ULTRASONIC DIFFERENTIAL DIAGNOSIS OF TUMORS

ULTRASONIC DIFFERENTIAL DIAGNOSIS OF TUMORS

Edited by

George Kossoff, D. Sc. Eng.
Director, Ultrasonics Institute
Sydney, N.S.W.
Australia

Morimichi Fukuda, M.D.
Associate Professor, Department of Internal Medicine
Sapporo Medical College
Sapporo, Japan

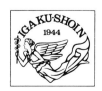

IGAKU-SHOIN   New York • Tokyo

Text Design by Eileen Ginsberg.
Typesetting by Maryland Composition Company, Inc. in Century Schoolbook.
Printing and Binding by Haddon Craftsmen, Inc.
Cover Design by Sybil Rubin Graphic Design.

Published and distributed by

IGAKU-SHOIN Ltd.,
5-24-3 Hongo, Bunkyo-ku, Tokyo

IGAKU-SHOIN Medical Publishers, Inc.,
1140 Avenue of the Americas, New York, N.Y. 10036

Library of Congress Cataloging in Publication Data
Main entry under title:

Ultrasonic differential diagnosis of tumors.

 Includes index.
 1. Cancer—Diagnosis. 2. Diagnosis, Ultrasonic.
3. Diagnosis, Differential. I. Kossoff, George.
II. Fukuda, Morimichi, 1929- . [DNLM: 1. Neoplasms—
Diagnosis. 2. Ultrasonics—Diagnostic use. 3. Diagnosis,
Differential. QZ 241 U463]
RC270.U47 1983 616.99′407543 83-174

ISBN: 0-89640-093-X

Printed and bound in the United States of America

10 9 8 7 6 5 4 3 2 1

CONTRIBUTORS

Yutaka Atomi, M.D.
First Department of Surgery
Faculty of Medicine
University of Tokyo
Tokyo, Japan

**David Arthur Carpenter,
M. Eng. Sc.**
Ultrasonics Institute
Sydney, N.S.W., Australia

**David O. Cosgrove, M.A., M.Sc.,
M.R.C.P.**
Royal Marsden Hospital, Sutton
Surrey, United Kingdom

Joan Croll, M.B., B.S.
The Sydney Square Diagnostic
    Breast Clinic
Sydney Square, Australia

Floyd Dunn, Ph.D.
Bioacoustics Research Laboratory
University of Illinois
Urbana, Illinois

Morimichi Fukuda, M.D.
Department of Internal Medicine
Sapporo Medical College
Sapporo, Japan

Stephen A. Goss, Ph.D.
Ultrasound Research Division
Indianapolis Center for Advanced
    Research, Inc.
Indianapolis, Indiana

Kaye A. Griffiths, R.N.
Ultrasonics Institute
Sydney, N.S.W., Australia

Sumio Inoue, M.D.
First Department of Surgery
Faculty of Medicine
University of Tokyo
Tokyo, Japan

Jack Jellins, B.Sc., B.E.
Ultrasonics Institute
Sydney, N.S.W., Australia

Nobuhiro Kawano, M.D.
First Department of Surgery
Faculty of Medicine
University of Tokyo
Tokyo, Japan

Tsugio Kitamura, M.D.
Ultrasound Laboratory
Center for Adult Diseases
Osaka, Japan

Takashi Koga, M.D.
Medical Corporation
Koga Hospital
Miyazaki, Japan

George Kossoff, D. Sc. Eng.
Ultrasonics Institute
Sydney, N.S.W., Australia

**Rod J. Lane, M.B., F.R.C.S.,
F.R.C.S.E., D.D.U., M.S.,
F.R.A.C.S.**
Sydney University
Department of Surgery
Royal North Shore Hospital
St. Leonards, N.S.W., Australia

George R. Leopold, M.D.
Division of Diagnostic Ultrasound
University of California
San Diego, California

Yasuhiko Morioka, M.D.
First Department of Surgery
Faculty of Medicine
University of Tokyo
Tokyo, Japan

David Nicholas, B.Sc., Ph.D., M.Inst.P.
Institute of Cancer Research
Royal Marsden Hospital, Sutton
Surrey, United Kingdom

Hiroshi Ohe, M.D.
Department of Urology
Kyoto Prefectural University of
Medicine
Kyoto, Japan

Richard H. Picker, M.B., B.S., F.R.A.C.O.G., Hon. F.R.A.C.R., D.D.U.
Section of Diagnostic Ultrasound
Royal North Shore Hospital
St. Leonards, N.S.W., Australia

Thomas S. Reeve, M.B., B.S.
Department of Surgery
Royal North Shore Hospital
St. Leonards, N.S.W., Australia

Arthur T. Rosenfield, M.D.
Department of Diagnostic Radiology
Yale University School of Medicine
Section of Ultrasound
Yale-New Haven Hospital
New Haven, Connecticut

Yasuaki Takehara, M.D.
Department of Diagnostic Imaging
Kanto Central Hospital
Tokyo, Japan

Hisaya Takeuchi, M.D.
Department of Obstetrics and
Gynecology
Juntendo University School of
Medicine
Tokyo, Japan

Sadanao Tane, M.D.
Department of Ophthalmology
St. Marianna University School of
Medicine
Kawasaki, Japan

Kenneth J. W. Taylor, M.D., Ph.D., F.A.C.P.
Department of Diagnostic Radiology
Yale University School of Medicine
Section of Ultrasound
Yale-New Haven Hospital
New Haven, Connecticut

Toshio Wagai, M.D.
Medical Ultrasonics Research
Center
Juntendo University School of
Medicine
Tokyo, Japan

Peter S. Warren, M.B., Ch.B., F.R.A.C.R., Dip. Obst., D.D.U.
Department of Diagnostic
Ultrasound
Royal Hospital for Women
Paddington, N.S.W., Australia

Hiroki Watanabe, M.D.
Department of Urology
Kyoto Prefectural University of
Medicine
Kyoto, Japan

Robert K. Zeman, M.D.
Abdominal Imaging Division
Department of Radiology
Georgetown University Hospital
Georgetown University Medical
School
Washington, D.C.

PREFACE

The imaging properties of ultrasonic B-mode equipment have been dramatically improved in the last few years. The axial and lateral resolution is beginning to approach the theoretical limits, and the contrast resolution has been refined to optimize the display of the internal texture of soft tissue organs. The performance characteristics of most static scanners today are similar, i.e., echograms of the same subject obtained with different equipment bear close resemblance. Real-time equipment is also firmly established, and its imaging characteristics are gradually beginning to match those of static scanners. Indeed, it would appear that a certain plateau in the quality of the imaging has been attained, and this suggests that the performance of conventional equipment is likely to remain relatively constant for the next few years.

The clinical use of B-mode ultrasound for the detection of localized and disseminated tumors in soft tissue organs is well established. Sufficient experience has now been gathered with high-quality instrumentation to determine on a statistical basis the sensitivity, specificity and accuracy of ultrasound diagnosis in the various applications. Although the technique cannot be used to identify tissue or to distinguish between benign and malignant tumors, the application of multiclassification criteria can frequently provide accurate information on the nature of the examined tissues, particularly when the results are taken in the context of the clinical history of the patient.

Despite the fact that the quality of the images provided by conventional B-mode equipment has reached a plateau, diagnostic ultrasound is continuing its growth. New clinical applications continue to be discovered as the existing equipment is used in new ways. The development of special-purpose equipment, such as water-path, small-part, combined B-mode and Doppler and internal scanners is also creating new uses. To date, an ultrasonic examination is based on the qualitative assessment of the information displayed on the echogram. Progress is being achieved in techniques that allow quantitative assessment of this data, and techniques for the measurement of other acoustic parameters of tissue are also beginning to open up many new areas of application.

With this in mind, we have invited some of the leading investigators in the field of ultrasonography to summarize the current status of ultrasonic differential diagnosis of tumors. The first four chapters describe the physical properties and principles that underlie the acquisition of ultrasonic images. The second and larger portion of the book is devoted to clinical examination of particular anatomical regions or functional systems. The examining technique, the choice of instrumentation, the multiclassification criteria and the results are documented. Because, as mentioned above, the imaging characteristics of the equipment are likely to remain relatively constant in the next few years, these descriptions will be current for some time to come. In part III, progress in tissue characterization and prospects for future developments are discussed. It is our intent that using this book the novice just entering the field will be able to determine the potential benefits of ultrasonic examinations and that established sonographers will be able to judge the efficacy of their procedures and, we hope, be encouraged to undertake new investigations. It is our goal to encourage the widespread use of high-quality ultrasonic diagnosis to advance the early detection of cancer.

George Kossoff
Morimichi Fukuda

CONTENTS

ULTRASONIC DIFFERENTIAL
DIAGNOSIS OF TUMORS

I
Basic Physics in Diagnostic Ultrasound

1

ULTRASONIC PROPERTIES OF TISSUES

Floyd Dunn

Stephen A. Goss

The fate of ultrasonic signals propagating within biological media is determined by the local acoustic (amplitude, frequency, etc.) and state (pressure, temperature, pathology, etc.) variables along the propagation pathway. Inasmuch as not all these quantities are measurable, at least not with usable accuracy and precision, compromises and accommodations must be reached and understood if the available data are to be applied to clinical procedures. The speed at which the signal travels in a tissue, the attenuation/absorption of the wave energy by the tissue and the features of the tissue responsible for reflection and scattering, generally subsumed in the concept of impedance, constitute the *ultrasonic propagation properties* of a tissue. These properties influence the obtaining of significant diagnostic ultrasound information and are important in producing and assessing biological effects. In this chapter the ultrasonic propagation properties of tissues that have been measured and reported (1, 2) are discussed and categorized.

SPEED

The speed of sound in tissues has been measured almost exclusively in vitro (1, 2). Figures 1 and 2 are graphic representations of data from in vivo and fresh in vitro tissue specimens in the 20–40°C temperature range, listed in order of increasing total protein and total collagen contents, respectively. The considerable range in the reported values likely is attributable to the use of different measuring methods, different specimen temperatures during measurement, different methods of specimen preparation and from different examples of specimens being chosen. The standard deviations range from less than 2% for brain, liver and kidney to approximately 7% for skin. Nevertheless, the data show that an ordering of tissue specimens in terms of increasing protein content is also an ordering for increasing speed of sound.

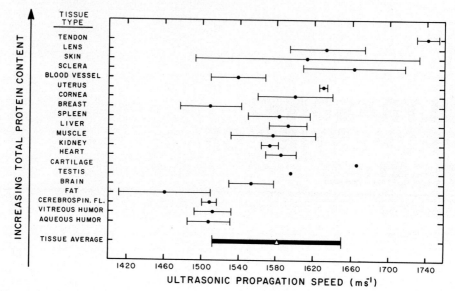

Figure 1. Ultrasonic propagation speed in tissues ordered by increasing total protein content. Data points indicate mean and bars standard deviation of reported measurements.

The ultrasonic velocity data compilation presented herein also enables an estimate to be made of the mean velocity among the 21 tissues for which results are available, though the use of such a mean value in applications other than where a gross estimate is required is not recommended (3, 4). Here, the mean ± standard deviation is 1581 ± 66 m/s which should be compared with the often quoted average ultrasonic velocity in tissue of 1540 m/s. Such estimates

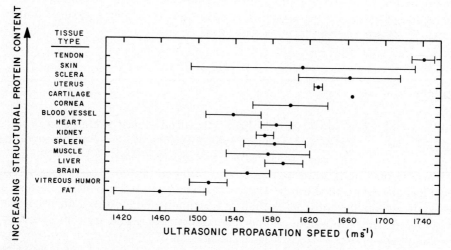

Figure 2. Ultrasonic propagation speed in tissues ordered by increasing structural protein content. Data points indicate mean and bars standard deviation of reported measurements.

should not replace velocity determination over the precise tissue path of interest, however, as the velocity among various soft tissues varies nearly 300 m/s.

ATTENUATION

Because parenchymal tissues conduct sound at approximately the same velocity as water, it has become customary to think of the soft tissues as liquidlike media having densities and compressibilities much like those of water but with significantly different attenuation and absorption properties, viz., much greater magnitudes and a nearly linear, rather than quadratic, dependence upon frequency. A considerable range of values has been reported (1, 2), apparently reflecting the difficulty in making and interpreting such measurements (5, 6), although methods of measurement and specimen preparations have improved with time and experience as published values have decreased (7). The reported attenuation range in some cases is more than 100%.

Figure 3 shows the ultrasonic attenuation coefficient for liver for in vivo and in vitro tissue specimens in the 20–40°C temperature range as a function of frequency. The figure includes all measurements reported up to early 1980. The mathematical expression and drawn straight line indicate the least-squares best fit for these data, where A is the attenuation coefficient (cm^{-1}), F is the frequency in megahertz and R indicates the goodness of fit ($R = 1$ for a perfect fit). Figures 4–6 show similar data for brain, muscle and fat.

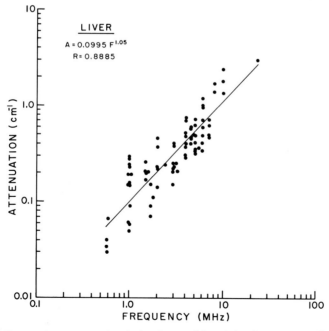

Figure 3. Ultrasonic attenuation in in vivo and fresh in vitro mammalian liver specimens in the temperature range 20–40°C as a function of frequency.

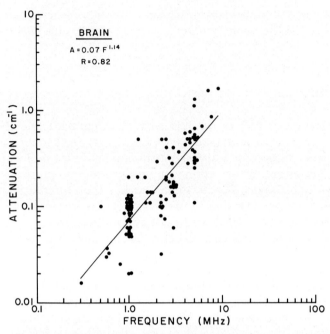

Figure 4. Ultrasonic attenuation in in vivo and fresh in vitro mammalian brain specimens in the temperature range 20–40°C as a function of frequency.

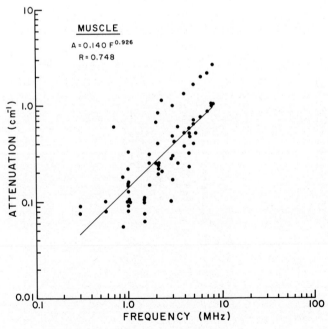

Figure 5. Ultrasonic attenuation in in vivo and fresh in vitro mammalian muscle specimens, perpendicular and parallel to fiber direction, in the temperature range 20–40°C as a function of frequency.

6

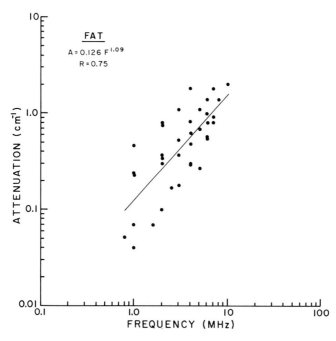

Figure 6. Ultrasonic attenuation in in vivo and fresh in vitro mammalian fat in the temperature range 20–40°C as a function of frequency.

These data show that the frequency dependence of attenuation is nearly linear for the four rather distinct tissues over the 1–10 MHz frequency range. The magnitude of the attenuation coefficient, however, appears to depend somewhat more upon tissue type, with muscle and fat exhibiting attenuation magnitudes roughly twice that for brain (in the lower end of this frequency range). Inasmuch as the macrostructural characteristics of tissue (dimensions on the order of a wavelength of sound or larger) affect the degree to which scattering losses at a given frequency contribute to overall attenuation, attenuation in heterogeneous tissues might be expected to be higher than in more homogeneous ones.

ABSORPTION

Few methods are available for measuring absorption directly (6). The transient thermoelectric method has been employed for studying freshly excised tissues as a function of frequency (8), and the results of such studies are shown in Figure 7. The exponents on frequency vary from 1.02 to 1.08 among testis, kidney, heart, brain, liver and tendon, even though these tissues represent substantial differences in their structural and chemical compositions. It is to be noted, however, that very pronounced differences in the magnitudes of the absorption occur, viz., tendon being four to five times greater than liver, brain, heart and kidney, which in turn are about twice that of testis. It should be noted too that heart, brain and kidney have approximately 16–18% protein,

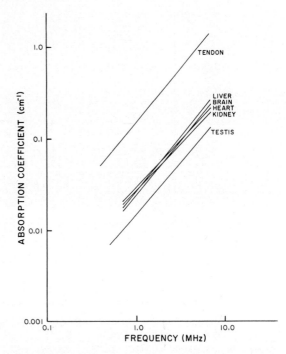

Figure 7. Frequency dependence of ultrasonic absorption in various tissues at 37°C (8). (From Goss SA, Frizzell LA, Dunn F: Ultrasonic absorption and attenuation in mammalian tissues. Ultrasound Med Biol 5: 181–186, 1979. Courtesy of Pergamon Press Ltd., Oxford.)

1–2% collagen and about 71–76% water. Tendon, on the other hand, has a total protein content of 35–40% with 30% collagen, but with a water content of only 63%. Testis has very little collagen, about 12% protein but has more than 80% water. (Testis may have a greater water content than any tissue other than fetal brain.) Though brain has lesser protein content than do kidney,

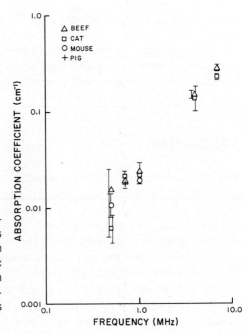

Figure 8. Species dependence of ultrasonic absorption in liver at 37°C. Bars represent standard deviation (8). (From Goss SA, Frizzell LA, Dunn F: Ultrasonic absorption and attenuation in mammalian tissues. Ultrasound Med Biol 5: 181–186, 1979. Courtesy of Pergamon Press Ltd., Oxford.)

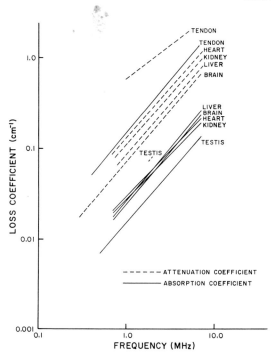

Figure 9. Comparison of ultrasonic attenuation and absorption in various tissues as a function of frequency (8). (From Goss SA, Frizzell LA, Dunn F: Ultrasonic absorption and attenuation in mammalian tissues. Ultrasound Med Biol 5: 181–186, 1979. Courtesy of Pergamon Press Ltd., Oxford.)

liver and heart, its greater lipid and lesser collagen contents may combine in some way to provide its similar absorption properties.

The species dependence of absorption for the single organ liver from beef, pig, cat and mouse, in the frequency range 0.5–7 MHz, all at 37°C is seen in Figure 8 to exhibit little, possibly negligible, difference in the observed values (8).

Comparison of these absorption measurements with the average published values for attenuation (1, 2) yields an interesting contrast (8), viz., that there is little difference between the frequency dependence of absorption and that of attenuation in the frequency range 0.5–7 MHz, suggesting that, whatever the source of differences in magnitude between attenuation and absorption values (i.e., scattering, reflection, measurement artifact, etc.), that mechanism is nearly linearly dependent upon frequency (Figure 9).

TEMPERATURE DEPENDENCE

Measurements of attenuation in excised tissues generally show decreasing attenuation temperature dependence with increasing temperature, as is expected of a fluid viscosity mechanism. However, the situation for in vivo absorption, which is the more pertinent quantity, may be considerably different. As it is very difficult to conduct observations as a function of temperature with an ordinary mammal, because of the superior temperature-controlling mechanism, measurements have been made using young mice, approximately 24 hours after birth, which are essentially poikilothermic animals (9, 10). The general demeanor of these studies is shown in Figure 10 where it is seen that

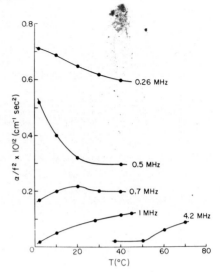

Figure 10. Frequency-free ultrasonic absorption in vivo in tissues as a function of frequency and temperature (9, 10).

the frequency-free absorption *vs* temperature comprises a family of curves whose maxima decrease and move toward ever increasing temperatures as a function of increasing frequency.

DEPENDENCE UPON CONSTITUENT MACROMOLECULES

It has long been known that the absorption of ultrasound in tissues is largely determined by the protein constituents (5) and, because of this, aqueous solutions of globular proteins have been studied as model systems of tissue wherein the tissue architecture may be relegated to, or associated with, the remaining portion of the attenuation (6). Most such studies have involved only globular proteins (different size/structure), which carry out the biochemical events in the physiological processes of the various organs. Studies of the ultrasonic properties of structural proteins in aqueous suspension have now been carried out (11) and it is pertinent to include these results with those of globular proteins and with tissues (12). Structural proteins provide a framework maintaining tissue structure integrity. It is to be noted that tissues comprised mainly of these proteins, mostly collagen, have much different elastic properties than do tissues having little collagen or are predominately comprised of globular protein. Figure 11 shows the values for the ultrasonic velocity of various tissues, as a function of the wet weight percentage of total protein, where the total protein content of the tissue is assumed to be in the form of globular protein and collagen. The upper and lower lines of Figure 11 describe the dependence of velocity for the globular and for the structural protein fractions of the total protein content each equal to zero, respectively (12). Accordingly, tissues predominately comprised of globular protein are expected to exhibit ultrasonic velocities near the value for collagen-free media, with a tissue wholly so constituted exhibiting that value for a solution of globular protein at the specified concentration. Similarly, collagenous tissues, such as tendon,

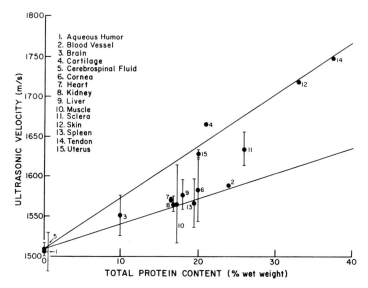

Figure 11. Dependence of ultrasonic velocity (1 MHz) on tissue proteins. Tissue measurements (●) are compared with the globular protein-free curve (upper curve) and the collagen-free curve (lower curve) (11). (From Goss SA, Frizzell LA, Dunn F, et al: Dependence of the ultrasonic properties of biological tissue on constituent proteins. J Acoust Soc Am 67: 1041–1044, 1980. Courtesy of American Institute of Physics.)

where a substantial fraction of the protein is in the form of collagen, are expected to exhibit values well above the collagen-free, globular protein value. This is borne out (Figure 11) in that liver, kidney, heart and muscle, all with approximately the same total protein, about 17%, of which very little, less than 1%, is collagen, have nearly the same velocities and appear near the collagen-free value for their wet weight percentage of total protein. Tendon, which is largely collagen (37.6% protein, 85% of which is collagen) exhibits the collagen value for its wet weight percentage of total protein. Fatty tissues contain little protein and their velocities are less than the others. Thus, it appears that the ultrasonic velocity in tissues is governed, in some way, by the ultrasonic properties of the individual macromolecular constituents comprising them.

Ultrasonic absorption appears to be governed by similar relationships. The absorption by tissues of sound at 1 MHz is seen in Figure 12 to fall between the values, at the appropriate wet weight percent of total protein, of the absorption of solutions of globular proteins in the 5–40% concentration range and of the absorption of suspensions of collagen in the 0.07–3.7% concentration range.

Thus, it appears that absorption in tissues is a linear superposition of the absorption properties of their protein constituents, and tissues appear, at least to a first approximation, to be composite materials whose ultrasonic properties are governed by the individual ultrasonic properties of their structural and globular protein contents.

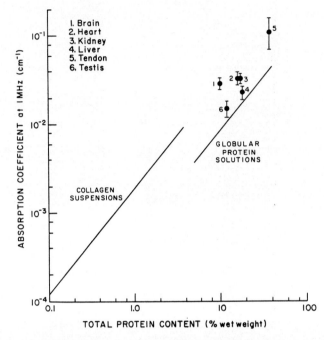

Figure 12. Dependence of ultrasonic absorption (1 MHz) on tissue proteins. Tissue measurements (●) appear between the curves defining the ultrasonic absorption of globular protein solutions and of collagen suspensions (11). (From Goss SA, Frizzell LA, Dunn F, et al: Dependence of the ultrasonic properties of biological tissue on constituent proteins. J Acoust Soc Am 67: 1041–1044, 1980. Courtesy of American Institute of Physics.)

SUMMARY

The data presented above indicate that the ultrasonic propagation properties of tissues are governed to some extent by their biochemical compositions and that substantial differences exist between reported values of attenuation and absorption coefficients of tissues, though nearly linear frequency dependence prevails in most tissues for both.

Future detailed measurements possibly will allow assignment of resolvably unique values to each tissue structure, including useful differentiable values for pathological states, so that attenuation, velocity and impedance values, as a function of state and of acoustic parameters, media, etc., should uniquely specify tissues for diagnostic purposes. It clearly is not necessary to have acoustic methods for discriminating between, say, brain and liver, but some diseased tissues that have a composition differing distinctly from that of surrounding tissues could be identifiable by such methods. For example, cirrhosis of the liver, as manifested by collagen deposited in place of normal tissues, should be easily identified, and is. However, metastases of, say, nerve tissue neoplasm in liver probably are not identifiable, at least in the early stages before cirrhosis of the liver tissue begins. A major problem of prediction, at present, is the paucity of data on abnormal tissues.

ACKNOWLEDGMENT

The authors gratefully acknowledge partial support for portions of the research described herein by grants from the National Institutes of Health.

REFERENCES

1. Goss SA, Johnston RL, Dunn F: Comprehensive compilation of empirical ultrasonic properties of mammalian tissues. J Acoust Soc Am 64: 423–457, 1978.
2. Goss SA, Johnston RL, Dunn F: Compilation of empirical ultrasonic properties of mammalian tissues II. J Acoust Soc Am 68: 93–108, 1980.
3. Rose JL, Goldberg BB: Basic Physics in Diagnostic Ultrasound. New York, Wiley, 1979.
4. McDicken WN: Diagnostic Ultrasonics, 2nd Ed. New York, Wiley, 1981.
5. Dunn F, O'Brien, Jr. WD, (eds): Ultrasonic Biophysics. Vol. 7, Benchmark Papers in Acoustics. Stroudsburg, Dowden, Hutchinson, & Ross, 1976, 410 pp.
6. Dunn F, Edmonds PD, Fry WJ: Absorption and dispersion of ultrasound in biological media. In Schwan HP (ed): Biological Engineering. New York, McGraw-Hill Book Co., 1969, pp 205–332.
7. Goss SA, Johnston RL, Dunn F: Ultrasound mammalian tissue properties literature search. Acoust Lett 1: 171–172, 1978.
8. Goss SA, Frizzell LA, Dunn F: Ultrasonic absorption and attenuation in mammalian tissues. Ultrasound Med Biol 5: 181–186, 1979.
9. Dunn F, Brady JK: Pogloshchenie Ul'trazvyeka V Biologicheskikh Sredakh (Ultrasonic absorption in biological media). (in Russian with English Abstr.) Biofizika 18: 1063–1066, 1973. English transl.: Biophysics 18: 1128–1132, 1974.
10. Dunn F, Brady JK: Temperature and frequency dependence of ultrasonic absorption in tissue. In Proceedings of the 8th International Congress on Acoustics. Trowbridge. Goldcrest Press, 1974, Vol 1, p 366c.
11. Goss SA, Frizzell LA, Dunn F, et al: Dependence of the ultrasonic properties of biological tissue on constituent proteins. J Acoust Soc Am 67: 1041–1044, 1980.
12. Goss SA, Dunn F: Ultrasonic propagation properties of collagen. Phys Med Biol 25: 827–837, 1980.

2

ULTRASONIC INSTRUMENTATION USED FOR TUMOR DIAGNOSIS

David Arthur Carpenter

In any ultrasonic diagnostic procedure it is important to use the most suitable instrument in the correct mode of operation and to ensure that it is producing the highest quality output. In ultrasonic tumor diagnosis, especially, where the differences between malignant and benign or normal tissue is often very small, both the technical capability of the instrument and the competence of the operator must be of the highest order.

Ultrasonic instrumentation used for tumor diagnosis can be divided into four main areas:

1) The modes of operation of the instrument, such as A-, B-, and M-modes and Doppler techniques.
2) The scan types, such as static or real-time, contact or water coupling, simple or compound scan.
3) The transducer effects, such as resolution, sensitivity, shadowing and enhancement.
4) The image processing, such as the electronic signal processing and the image recording techniques used.

MODES OF OPERATION

The A-mode scan, which simply displays echo amplitude against time (i.e. penetration) for a given line of sight, has little application in modern grey scale equipment. In bistable and early grey scale equipment it was useful in determining whether an area of low level echoes was really echo free (cystic lesion) or had very low echoes (fat or pus). With modern grey scale equipment this determination can be made directly from the B-mode image. The use of A-mode in direct diagnosis is restricted to applications such as locating a midline shift in the brain.

14

A new application of A-mode scanning has emerged: the recording of a line of echoes for computer analysis. Various digital processing techniques can be used for resolution enhancement and tissue characterization. They can elucidate such characteristics as the attenuation, velocity, echo-scattering cross section and movement patterns for a given area of tissue.

The M-mode technique, in which the movement of interfaces is plotted against time for a given line of sight, is used mainly for the diagnosis of cardiac or related diseases. An experienced operator can determine valve conditions, such as stenosis or vegetation, and wall conditions, such as ischemia and pericardial effusion. Research is being carried out with M-mode as a technique for diagnosing diseases of the vascular system, such as aortic aneurysms and carotid and occular vessel disease.

With the advent of high-quality, B-mode real-time scanners, a number of cardiac conditions previously diagnosed with M-mode are now being detected with real-time scanning or a combination of the two modalities. Real-time investigation is ideally suited to conditions such as atrial myxomia and septal defects. The mechanically scanned or phased-array sector scanners are most suited to cardiac examination because of the small ultrasonic window available through the intercostal spaces and under the costal margin.

Many real-time units have the ability to give a simultaneous M mode readout along one or more lines of sight selected by the operator, and some units now have a pulsed Doppler system for blood flow measurements within the heart.

The B mode or two-dimensional scan is by far the most commonly used for ultrasound diagnosis, and the instrumentation comes in numerous configurations. Wide clinical acceptance and considerable technical development in recent years have brought most B-mode scanners to a uniformly high standard of performance. This does not imply that tumor diagnosis is always easy with current equipment. Sometimes two or three types of scanner or scanning technique can be used without obtaining a definitive diagnosis. The various types of equipment and processing developments are discussed in the following sections.

The Doppler technique (1) does not use a pulse-echo system to image tissue interfaces in the same way as the A-, B-, or M-mode. It detects the velocity of moving interfaces by measuring the frequency shift of the returned echo signal. This frequency shift (called the Doppler shift after its discoverer) is commonly used to calculate the velocity of moving heart walls or blood flow velocity in the arterial and venous circulation. The simplest systems use continuous-wave ultrasound to detect fetal heart movement and the blood velocity in superficial vessels. Because they use continuous-wave sound, these systems do not give any range (i.e., depth) information as to the source of the Doppler shifted signal. The more complex systems (called pulsed Doppler systems) use a short burst of ultrasound, and the return signal is gated to register only the signal from a specific depth as set by the range gate. If this pulsed Doppler system is combined with a B-mode scanner, which will give the area of the vessel and the angle of approach of the beam to the vessel, it is possible to measure both the velocity and the flow rate of blood (2).

It is also possible to image vessels using a Doppler system by systematically moving the probe over the vessel of interest (e.g., the carotid artery) and setting up the electronics to only write a line on the screen when blood flow is detected. Hence, clots, plaques or occlusions will show up as a narrowing or complete loss of signal from the vessel.

SCAN TYPES

B-mode scanners fall into the two main categories of static scanners and real-time units. The static scanner of the contact or waterbath type can provide an overall view of an area such as the upper abdomen and can give both a compound and a simple scan of the area. High-quality results with the contact scanner depend to some degree on the operator, and both types require a few seconds to complete a scan and to move from one scan plane to another. For this reason, any movement of the scanned area can blur or distort the image. The real-time scanner overcomes this by operating at a rate of more than 20 scans per second, and it is rapidly positioned on the optimum scan plane. It has the drawback of some loss of quality due to the restricted number of lines of sight imposed by the rapid acquisition rate, but the quality difference relative to static scanners is minimized in the latest equipment (3). The real-time units provide only a simple scan image with a limited field or "keyhole" view of an organ being scanned. The ideal setup would be a static scanner and a real-time unit. Recently, an instrument called the small-parts scanner has become commercially available. These usually are of the waterbath type and operate at higher frequencies (5–10 MHz) to produce high-resolution scans of the superficial areas of the body. They are ideally suited for the breast, thyroid, carotid, testis and eye and for head and abdominal examination of the neonate.

The waterbath scanner offers advantages for scanning lesions in deformable organs such as the breast or testis by providing a uniform scan rate and the possibility of a series of scans. It provides a stable, accurately defined scan plane for rescanning an area and defining a line of sight for other measurements, such as velocity or attenuation in tissue. Also, with this instrument there is little restriction on transducer size. Large apertures for high resolution with fixed-focus or annular-array transducers can be used (4).

The contact scanner can offer more angulation of the transducer than the waterbath type for scanning under the costal margin or deep into the pelvis. For ultrasonically guided needle biopsy, one of course is restricted to a contact or real-time scanner.

The real-time scanner comes in a number of configurations, with a mechanically moved transducer, a fixed transducer with a mechanically moved mirror or an electronically scanned beam from an array of transducer elements (5). There are considerable differences between the beam patterns for different real-time units. The mechanically scanned units technically are very similar to a conventional contact scanner and, therefore, offer similar performance levels, whereas the transducer arrays have some unique properties, which will be discussed in the section, Transducer Effects. The scan format is either rectangular or sector, with most units being of the skin-contact type. The sector scanner is more suited to areas of limited access, such as the heart, pelvis and neonatal head, whereas rectangular format instruments, such as the linear array scanners, are best used for more general upper abdominal and obstetrical and gynecological applications, where a wider field of view is needed for structures close to the transducer. There are some mechanically scanned real-time units that give an annular scan that is fairly wide at the skin surface (on the order of 6–8 cm) and expands to a wider scan with depth, similar to the sector format.

All real-time units have had the disadvantage of a limited number of lines of sight available per scan due to the necessity of operating at high scan rates. This was particularly true of the sector format, where the lines diverge with increasing depth to give a very sparse line spacing on posterior structures. With the digital scan convertor it is possible to linearly interpolate between the scan lines. This is justified by the transducer beamwidth, which is considerably wider than the line spacing. This feature, which gives a uniform display over the whole scan area, is now available on a number of real-time units.

The advent of grey scale and real-time scanning has caused an increase in the use of simple scans, but simple and compound scanning are complementary in defining lesions (6).

The compound scan gives better definition of boundary structures around organs and the echograms are closer in appearance to an anatomical slice. The resolution of a structure can vary in a simple scan, depending on the structure's orientation to the ultrasound beam, whereas a compound scan gives consistent resolution. The simple scan is superior for structures that are moving with respiration or cardiac pulsations because the movement is traced out on the scan. In a compound scan the motion causes blurring and resolution is lost. As will be discussed below, the simple scan is essential for displaying enhancement, shadowing and refraction effects behind structures.

TRANSDUCER EFFECTS

The transducer has been called the "eye" of an ultrasound system. The correct selection and optimum performance of the transducer are essential to obtaining maximum diagnostic information (7, 8) because transducer shortcomings can rarely be overcome by signal processing changes.

Transducers are designed for maximum resolution in both the axial (i.e., along the beam) and lateral (i.e., across the beam) directions (Figure 1). Axial resolution is determined by the length of the ultrasound pulse, and this is minimized in modern transducers by use of electrical loading and damping, mechanical backing and quarter-wave matching layers. The lateral resolution is defined by the width of the ultrasound beam and this can be reduced by the use of larger apertures and by focussing techniques (9). These techniques are limited in single-element transducers in which the range of focus (or depth of field) is reduced as the degree of focussing is increased.

An increase in frequency improves both axial and lateral resolution but does so at the cost of reduced penetration of the beam due to the increased attenuation of tissue at higher frequencies. In typical weakly focused transducers, axial resolution is three to five times better than lateral resolution, and use

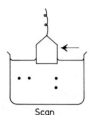

Scan

B-mode Display

Figure 1. Scanning of targets to define lateral resolution (one target next to the other) and axial resolution (one target behind the other).

should be made of this whenever possible. For example, in scanning small vessels such as the superior mesenteric artery, carotid artery or common bile duct, one should use a simple scan in the longitudinal plane, keeping the beam approximately normal to the vessel (Figure 2) so that the vessel walls are displayed with optimum resolution and do not encroach on the interior of the vessel.

Poor lateral resolution can cause false low-level echoes to be displayed in liquid-filled areas such as vessels and gallbladder as a result of energy returned from areas adjacent to the area central to the beam (Figure 3). Similarly, calculi may not shadow because the beam is too wide (10, 11).

The effects known as shadowing or enhancement are produced when the area being scanned attenuates the ultrasound beam more or less than the surrounding tissues for which the time-gain compensation of the echoscope has been adjusted. Hence, a lower echo level is returned to the transducer from the structures behind an area of high attenuation, and on the display a shadow appears to be cast on the posterior structures (Figure 4). Similarly, an area of low attenuation appears to enhance the echo levels behind it (6).

A simple scan is used to demonstrate these effects because the shadowing or enhancement will be overwritten in a compound scan. These effects can provide valuable diagnostic information because many lesions produce defined attenuation relative to normal areas, such as liver parenchyma or glandular

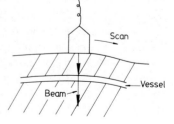

Scan

Vessel

Beam

Figure 2. Scanning a vessel at right angles to the ultrasound beam to make use of the better axial resolution of the transducer.

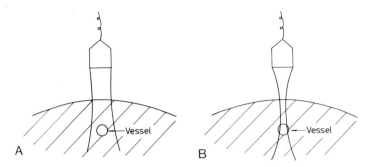

Figure 3. Beamwidth Effects. In *A* the small vessel may not be adequately displayed due to the wide beam producing echoes from the surrounding tissue.

tissue of the breast. For instance, enhancement behind an echo-free area is a stronger indication of a cystic lesion than is the simple lack of internal echoes.

Reflective and refractive bending of the ultrasound beam due to velocity differences between the fluid and the surrounding tissue (12) cause shadowing behind certain tumors that produce high attenuation (Figure 4) and behind the edges of larger liquid-filled areas, such as a cyst or gallbladder.

As greater dynamic range and more multielement transducers such as linear arrays, sector-phased arrays or annular arrays are used in echoscopes, spurious emissions and unwanted resonance modes, problems not encountered with a well-designed single-element circular transducer, are becoming more important. These may take the form of sidelobes caused by edge effects on small array elements or grating lobes caused by phasing effects between elements. These unwanted lobes on the beam pattern mean that small amounts of energy are transmitted in and received from directions other than that of the main beam of the transducer. Also, in small array elements, resonance modes other than the normal thickness mode may be excited and add to the transducer output. When one scans from a highly reflective boundary layer between organs into an area of little or no echo return, the sidelobes from the main beam can reproduce echoes of lower amplitude from the strong reflector. These are

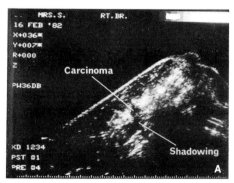
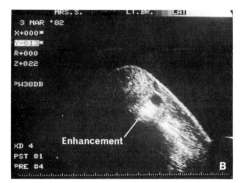

Figure 4. Example of (*A*) shadowing behind an infiltrating duct carcinoma of the breast and (*B*) enhancement behind a cyst.

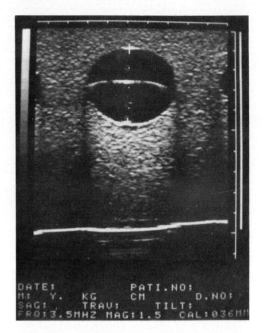

Figure 5. A sidelobe artifact displayed on each side of a point reflector within the echo-free area of a tissue phantom scanned by a linear-array transducer.

displayed as artifacts in the lower level region (Figure 5). These spurious echoes give indistinct boundaries and low-level signals in areas of the scan that should be echo free, resulting in what has been described as a "mushy" appearance.

Sector-phased arrays are more prone to these problems than linear arrays, because the sector arrays generally use smaller elements and have more phasing delays introduced to steer and focus the beam. These transducer effects are reduced in the latest units by careful design and uniform construction of array elements. The sector array is particularly suited to cardiac applications, where its high scan rate and small transducer size is an advantage over other real-time scanners.

IMAGE PROCESSING

Diagnosis with B-mode depends on recognition of anatomical relationships between organs and tissue texture within organs. This is a matter of pattern recognition and is still largely qualitative. A large amount of research and development in instrumentation has been aimed at various types of image processing to improve the diagnostic value of this pattern recognition process. Recently, computing techniques have been employed to extract quantitative information from the scan in the form of parameters such as attenuation, velocity and movement of tissue.

The original method of producing grey scale ultrasound images used a nonlinear compression amplifier to compress the dynamic range of the echoes, which were integrated onto film by an open-shutter camera technique. An even scanning rate and considerable operator skill were necessary if parts of the image were not to be overwritten. With the advent of the analogue scan convertor, there was a rapid increase in the clinical use of ultrasound, because this instrument could store the image in a peak detection (or equilibrium writing) mode. The peak value of the echo at each point in the scan was stored and values were not integrated up at a point. In this way overwriting was largely removed. The analogue scan converter could also operate in the integrate mode, and its greater input dynamic range capability as compared with direct film recording often allowed a selection of compression curves (preprocessing) before the image was stored. By varying the compression curve one can spread a particular tissue, such as liver parenchyma, over a greater grey scale range, allowing homogeneous lesions to be more easily detected. Some postprocessing also was available, because the gamma curve could be varied, the image could be zoomed up in size, and certain echo ranges could be highlighted as the image was read out to the television monitor. Although excellent image quality was available, the analogue storage tube suffered defocussing and aging problems and was too slow during erase to be used for real-time applications.

Virtually all current instruments use a digital scan convertor (13) as their primary image-processing and storage system. The echo level at each point in the scan is processed and stored as a number in a digital memory from where it can be read out in television format to the image recording system, which may be a polaroid or multiformat camera or a video disc or tape system. The digital scan convertor memory is usually arranged with 512 × 512 pixels (or picture elements) and 16 or 32 grey levels for each pixel (14).

A wide range of preprocessing compression curves is available and integration or peak detection storage can be used. Another mode, called "survey," can be selected. In this mode each new line of echoes replaces the previous one in the memory so that the image continually is updated as the scan proceeds. This clearly is useful for real-time applications.

The degree of variability in postprocessing functions normally is greater with the digital scan convertor.

The peak detection process retains the strongest echo in each picture element, and, hence, the specular boundary echoes are emphasized. Organ parenchyma appears speckled with higher level echoes. The beamwidth effect can be seen on large specular echoes, and this may obliterate smaller detail.

The integration process can be improved by dividing the sum of the echoes in each pixel by the number of echoes to obtain an average value. This removes the overwriting problem associated with straight integration without abolishing the resolution improvement that this technique can offer. In compound scans the beam edges are reduced when a reflector is scanned from a number of different directions. Specular reflectors are less prominent than with a peak detected image, and the speckle pattern of the tissue texture is a more uniform grey.

The choice of peak or integrate (or average) processing can depend on the type of scan and the organ being investigated. Peak may be suited to scans of homogeneous tissue, such as the liver, whereas integrate (or average) may reduce the specular reflectors and show up finer details in compound scans, such as those of the breast and of fetal structures (15) (Figure 6).

Average processing requires more computing capability than that possessed

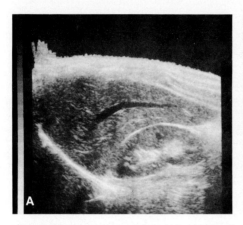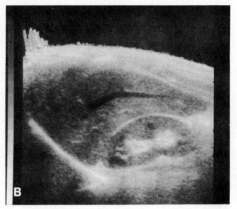

Figure 6. Types of image-processing techniques: (A) peak detection, (B) average processing.

by the digital scan convertors presently on the market, but some manufacturers are considering the introduction of these facilities.

The other processing modality that is feasible by modern digital techniques is the measurement of tissue parameters such as attenuation rate, movement and velocity (16, 17), a technique that will prove extremely important in defining a discrete tumor and in diagnosing disseminated conditions such as fatty infiltration. These processes are still in the research stage, but most digital scan convertors can select a given pixel or area of scan and read out the stored echo level, which can help in comparing the echo levels of different organs (e.g., liver and pancreas).

CONCLUSIONS

Although the performance of most current pulse-echo instruments consistently is of high quality, it still is important that the most suitable instrument for a particular scan be selected and that it be operated in a competent manner. Instruments must be standardized regularly and operators must be adequately trained if maximum diagnostic information is to be obtained. Current instruments still are basically only simple displays of impedance discontinuities, and developments in areas such as array transducers, Doppler blood flow measurements and digital image processing will continue to improve the capability of ultrasonic instrumentation in tumor diagnosis.

REFERENCES

1. Gill RW: Doppler ultrasonic bloodflow measurement. Australasian Bulletin of Medical Physics and Biophysics 71: 30–39, 1977.
2. Gill RW: Pulsed Doppler with B-mode imaging for quantitative blood flow measurement. Ultrasound Med Biol 5: 223–235, 1979.

3. Kossoff G: The king is dead long live the king. Australas Radiol 24: 220, 1980.

4. Kossoff G: Automated ultrasonic scanning techniques. In Kurjak A (ed): Recent Advances in Ultrasound Diagnosis. Amsterdam, Excerpta Medica, 1978, pp 22–35.

5. Wilkinson RW: Principles of real-time two-dimensional B-scan ultrasonic imaging. J Med Eng Technol 5: 21–29, 1981.

6. Kossoff G, Garrett WJ, Carpenter DA, et al: Principles and classification of soft tissue by grey scale echography. Ultrasound Med Biol 2: 89–105, 1976.

7. Carpenter DA: Ultrasonic transducers. In Wells PNT and Ziskin MC (Eds): Clinics in Diagnostic Ultrasound, Vol 5. New York, Churchill Livingstone Press, 1980, Chapt 3.

8. Kossoff G: The ultrasonic transducer. Int Ophthalmol Clin 9: 523–541, 1969.

9. Kossoff G: Analysis of focusing action of spherically curved transducers. Ultrasound Med Biol 5: 359–365, 1979.

10. Filly RA, Moss AA, May LW: In vitro investigation of gallstone shadowing with ultrasound tomography. J Clin Ultrasound 7: 255–262, 1979.

11. Sommer FG, Taylor KJW: Differentiation of acoustic shadowing due to calculi and gas collections. Radiol 135: 399–403, 1981.

12. Robinson DE, Wilson LW, Kossoff G: Shadowing and enhancement in ultrasonic echograms by reflection and refraction. J Clin Ultrasound 9: 181–188, 1981.

13. Carpenter DA, Robinson DE, Kossoff G: Digital and Analog Scan Converters for Ultrasound Imaging. Recent Advances in Ultrasound Diagnosis Amsterdam, Excerpta Medica, 1980, p 67.

14. Ophir J: Digital scan converters in diagnostic ultrasound imaging. Proc IEEE 67: 654–664, 1979.

15. Robinson DE, Knight PC: Computer reconstruction techniques in compound scan pulse echo imaging. Ultrasonic Imaging 3: 217–234, 1981.

16. Wilson LS, Robinson DE: Ultrasonic measurement of small displacements and deformations of tissue. Ultrasonic Imaging 4: 71–82, 1982.

17. Robinson DE, Chen T, Wilson LS: Measurement of velocity of propagation from ultrasonic pulse echo data. Ultrasound Med Biol 8: 413–420, 1982.

3

PRESENT STATUS OF ULTRASONIC TISSUE CHARACTERIZATION

David Nicholas

Over the past decade the meaning of the term "tissue characterization" has become somewhat unspecific within the field of ultrasonic diagnosis. Unfortunately, this has led many clinicians to regard this research activity as one which provides information of interest only to physicists and engineers by means unrelated to medical diagnosis. Therefore, it is important to emphasize that these new techniques and concepts are related to older ultrasonic diagnostic procedures. In its simplest form, tissue characterization is the identification of parameters relating to a tissue that are well correlated with the type or condition of that tissue. This implies that traditional visual interpretation of ultrasonic images is also a form of tissue characterization, albeit a subjective one. In this chapter I will briefly describe work done within this field, emphasizing interrelationships between the various techniques and existing diagnostic procedures. Most of the work has been conducted in the laboratory with excised tissues or phantoms, but only those techniques that have resulted in clinical trials will be discussed here. Readers are urged also to consult review articles (1–4) for a broader discussion of this topic.

The number of physical parameters considered appropriate for the ultrasonic characterization of human soft tissues has increased as our fundamental understanding and technology have developed. The possibility of noninvasively identifying local abnormalities in tissue was foreseen in some of the earliest diagnostic work (5), and tissue characterization using sound waves was explored as long ago as 1939 by Pohlmann (6). It is only in the past few years, however, that such techniques have achieved a more quantitative application and attracted the attention of diagnosticians.

I will present my discussion in four parts (Table 1) that are analogous to the chronological development of diagnostic ultrasound. The first section deals with the use of simple pulse-echo, A-scan data for simple quantitation of the visual appearance and for deriving information pertaining to the bulk acoustic properties of the tissue. The discussion of parameterization and enhancement of B-mode echograms in second section extends the information into two dimensions. An adjunct to this section has to do with the use of diffraction techniques for investigating the orientation dependence of scattering from small

24

TABLE 1. Current Approaches to Ultrasonic Tissue Characterization In Vivo.

A-Scan-Related Techniques
A-scan pattern recognition
Bulk property measurements: frequency dependence of attentuation
                               average frequency dependence of backscatter
Structural assessment of backscatter: spectral interference effects
                               impediography
B-scan Techniques
B-scan pattern recognition and feature extraction
B-scan image enhancement
Orientation dependence of backscattering (diffraction)
Tissue Dynamics
Pulsed Doppler methods
Time-dependent diffraction scanning
A-scan correlation analysis
Other Techniques
Attenuation and velocity reconstruction (through transmission)
Backscatter reconstruction.
Holography ⎫
Transmission imaging ⎬ not presently used for tissue characterization

tissue volumes. This aspect extends into the third part, where the dynamic aspects of tissue imaging are considered. The techniques that make use of a nonstandard data-gathering system, such as transmission imaging and computerized tomography, are discussed in the concluding section.

A-SCAN-RELATED TECHNIQUES

The advent of grey scale imaging techniques in pulse-echo ultrasound (7) resulted in exploitation of the specific values of echo intensity for characterizing various tissue types. Kossoff et al (8) have listed tissue types that can be characterized by the relative echo intensities displayed on the B-scan image. Taylor (9) reported that other features of the displayed image, such as "shadowing," can also aid in the differentiation of focal abnormalities. Furthermore, similar empirical approaches have long been used in ophthalmology for classifying orbital disease by observation of the rate of reduction of A-scan amplitude within the tissue (10, 11).

A more quantitative analysis of the A-scan was first attempted by Mountford and Wells (12, 13), who used off-line techniques to distinguish cirrhotic from normal hepatic tissue. Their findings suggested that although the rate of reduction of the A-scan with distance into the tissue was similar for both tissue types, differentiation could still be achieved when the overall intensities of the waveforms were compared. This finding has been confirmed subjectively in many clinical studies (14, 15) and has provided a useful aid to hepatic diagnosis. Recently, Lerski et al (16) have used more sophisticated techniques to analyze a variety of characteristics revealed by the shape of the A-scan. Using six features extracted from the A-scan, they have obtained an accuracy of 74% in discriminating among normal, fatty, alcoholic hepatitic and cirrhotic conditions of liver tissue.

Although such techniques are diagnostically useful, they fail to separate the two basic factors, attenuation and spatial variation in scattering strength, that contribute to A-scan information. To a first-order approximation, the rate of decrease of echo strength with distance into the tissue provides a measure of the bulk attenuating properties of the tissue. In B-scanning this factor can usually be eliminated (to a first-order approximation) by judicious use of "time-gain compensation." However, it has been suggested (17, 18) that the bulk attenuating properties of a tissue may be characteristic of its pathological condition. Although much work has been performed on the attenuation characteristics of excised tissues (as summarized by Goss et al [19]), little effort has been made to discover the attenuation coefficients of tissues in vivo. Kuc (20) and Lizzi et al (21) have contributed to our knowledge in this area by

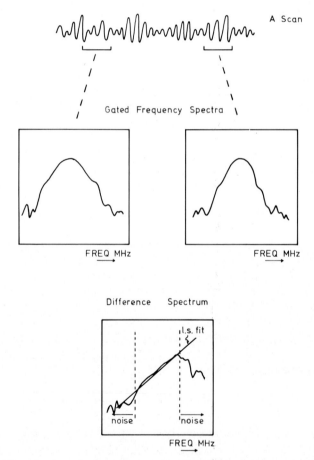

Figure 1. Schematic representation of the evaluation of the frequency-dependent attenuation coefficient in vivo. (After Kuc R: Clinical application of an ultrasound attenuation coefficient estimation technique for liver pathology characterization. IEEE Trans Biomed Eng 27: 312–319, 1980.)

transforming information from the range-selected portions of the A-scan to the frequency domain. Comparison of averaged frequency spectra for specific depths into the tissue yields a frequency-dependent attenuation coefficient. Kuc (20) has studied hepatic tissue and derived his attenuation values from individual A-scans separated into time-limited sections (Figure 1). His findings show that inflamed livers produce lower than normal attenuation coefficient values (expressed in dB cm^{-1} MHz^{-1}) and cirrhotic livers yield higher than normal values. Lizzi and Coleman (22) achieved success in their estimates of orbital fat attenuation in situ (1.2 dB cm^{-1} MHz^{-1}).

Structural Assessment

It is generally accepted that the echoes returning to the transducer in a pulse-echo investigation are due to scattering within the tissue, and it therefore seems reasonable to suppose that the backscattered echoes depend upon the arrangement of scatterers within that tissue (18). Since it has been shown that attenuation in a tissue can depend upon acoustic frequency, it also seems reasonable to suspect that scattering, as a contributor to attenuation, may also depend upon frequency. In vitro studies with various soft tissues have illustrated this effect (23–26).

Clinical trials by Lizzi et al (21, 27) have shown that scattering information indicative of specific tissue structures can be extracted from the basic A-scan waveforms. The A-scan is electrically time-gated to select echoes originating from a preselected volume of tissue whose identity is determined by the delay and duration of the electronic gate and by the transducer beamwidth. The time-gated portion of the backscattered echo-train is fed into a scanning electronic spectrum analyzer, which displays the gated echo function in terms of its frequency spectrum. Comparison of the averaged frequency spectrum for the backscattered data with a reference spectrum has led the authors to classify tissue in terms of three parameters:

1) Absolute reflectance, referenced to a standard flat glass plate target
2) Frequency slope of backscattering strength (dB/MHz)
3) "Resonant" frequency (MHz).

The third spectral characteristic was employed primarily in the examination of retinal detachment. The scalloped spectrum obtained from a detached retina (Figure 2) is typical of spectra from well-defined thin membranes and is the result of interference between acoustic reflections from the anterior and posterior surfaces of the retina. The spacing of the spectral nulls directly relates to retinal thickness. Similar spectra have been reported (22) for retinas overlying choroidal tumors (e.g., malignant melanomas).

These measurements now provide direct information concerning the spatial relationship of scattering structures in tissue and as such relate to the anatomical variability associated with various disease conditions. Spectral studies have been performed by Sommer et al (28, 29) in investigating hepatic and splenic conditions. In these situations the tissue structures are spatially ar-

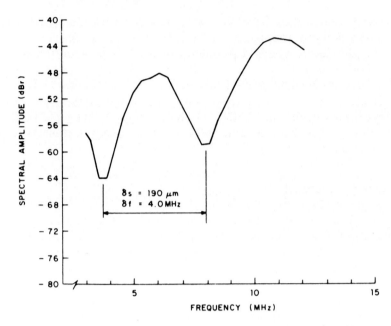

Figure 2.   Frequency spectrum from a detached retina. (From Lizzi FL, Laviola MA, Coleman DJ: Tissue signature characterization utilizing frequency domain characterization. Proceedings of the IEEE Ultrasonics Symposium. New York, IEEE, 1976, pp 714–719.)

ranged in a three-dimensional matrix and the spectral scalloping can only tentatively be related to actual structural separations. However, the results are encouraging and seem to permit a characterization of some disease states that are poorly diagnosed by conventional B-scan imaging.

In concluding this section I would like to comment on the reflection characteristics of tissue boundaries. Conventional imaging portrays such interfaces only in terms of the intensity of the reflected echoes. If, however, the original radio frequency information is examined, both the amplitudes and phases of the reflected echoes can be monitored. This information can be used to characterize the boundaries between two media of different acoustic impedance Z ($Z = \rho c$, where ρ is the density of the medium and c is the velocity of sound within the medium). Unfortunately, this technique (30, 31) has major limitations: it requires the tissue to conform to a layered medium and can only yield absolute values for impedance when the acoustic pulse impinges on a tissue interface at normal incidence. Despite these drawbacks, Jones (32) has used these measurements in vivo in characterizing orbital lesions and reports some success in characterizing differing tumor types. Figure 3 illustrates an impedance profile associated with these studies.

In reference to all these techniques, it must be emphasized that the A scan information used is that which contributes to the conventional video B scan image. No new echo information is created, rather a more quantitative interpretation is formulated from the conventional pulse-echo waveforms.

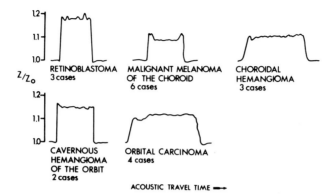

Figure 3. Typical impediograms for several orbital lesions. (From Jones JP: *In vivo* characterization of several lesions in the eye using ultrasonic impediography. In Metherell AF (ed): Acoustical Imaging Vol. 8, New York, Plenum Press, 1980, pp 539–546.)

B-SCAN TECHNIQUES

The information held in a full B-scan extends the A-scan into another dimension, implying that techniques applied to simple A-scans could have more powerful applications when extended to two dimensions, hence the recent growth of interest in applying image pattern and texture analysis to B-scans. The obvious drawbacks are the need for large data depositories, fast data capture and sophisticated computational facilities.

Two basic approaches have been adopted: an expensive on-line dedicated data acquisition system is used to collect each radio frequency echo A-scan (33) or existing video storage devices, analogue and/or digital scan conversion memories, are used as temporary storage for subsequent transfer (at slow data rates) to permanent computer storage (34). Although the latter technique is relatively simple and inexpensive, it is limited by the loss of all phase information originally present in the radio frequency signal. Furthermore, it also is affected by the preprocessing of the echo information before scan conversion (35).

Once the B-scan data are stored in a computer, two approaches are possible. Waag et al (36), for example, have carried out signal processing on B-scan data obtained from the heart and abdomen and have used "Fourier-domain filtering" to enhance certain image characteristics, such as structure boundaries. Other forms of filtering have been used by Wessels et al (37) to enhance characteristics of prostate lesions. These approaches are aimed at manipulating the original image to form an "enhanced" version that can be better visually interpreted.

Alternatively, one can implement two-dimensional feature-extraction algorithms similar to those reported for A-scan techniques. This topic has received considerable stimulation from applications in such fields as aerial photography and microbiology. Preliminary work by Nicholas et al (34) has indicated that hepatic lesions can be partially classified by quantitation of the amplitude and spatial characteristics they present on the video B-scan image. Lorenz et al (38), in a study of various hepatic diseases, both diffuse and focal, quote an overall accuracy of 70% with discriminant analysis based on 150 parameters calculated for each of the 597 images (135 subjects) collected. If one limits the discrimination to the diffuse hepatic diseases (cirrhosis, fatty infiltration and hepatitis) and normal tissue, the accuracy increases to approximately 73%. This accuracy has been confirmed in a separate study of 85 subjects by Nicholas et al (39).

These studies indicate that quantitation of images, with high-technology computing facilities providing the data extractions and anlaysis, can greatly aid our present subjective evaluation. The goal of such work will be the selection of a limited set of features and appropriate analysis that can be performed by a microprocessor. It then will be feasible to integrate such techniques into conventional ultrasonic imaging machines for on-line evaluation.

Structural Assessment

In the section on A-scan techniques I stressed that the spectral techniques currently used are limited to the assessment of tissue separations projected into the direction of the acoustic beam. Measurements performed in this manner accurately describe the true situation only when the structures either are aligned normal to the A-scan direction (as in ophthalmology) or are isotropically distributed as a truly homogeneous medium. If neither of these conditions are satisfied then an assessment in two dimensions will provide more accurate information.

Another experimental approach to deriving tissue structure information has been to record patterns of variation of echo intensity that occur with changes in the relative orientation between the tissue structure and the ultrasonic beam (40, 41) while working with a limited acoustic frequency bandwidth. Implementation of such an approach in vivo requires a purpose-built scanning arm (Figure 4) that directs the transducer at the same volume of tissue while performing an isocentric B-scan (42). The technique is equivalent to that of Lizzi and Coleman (22) described above, except only a narrow spectral bandwidth is investigated for the range of scanning motion. In initial clinical trials of this machine by Nicholas (43), the diffraction patterns associated with hepatic disease (Figure 5) yielded a 96% success rate in differentiating malignant, including 11 cases of diffuse infiltration, from normal liver tissue. The technique also showed promise in diagnosing other nonmalignant diffuse disorders such as cirrhosis and hepatitis. In a study of 52 patients with suspected thyroid disorders, Merton et al (44) were successful 88% of the time in discriminating among follicular adenomas, degenerating follicular adenomas and colloid masses.

It has been stressed (43) that the clinical value of this technique lies in its ability to empirically characterize various disease conditions even though it is incapable of providing an absolute structural assessment of tissues except where a degree of anisotrophy exists, as in skeletal muscle. Complete structural evaluation can be achieved only by performing a three-dimensional in-

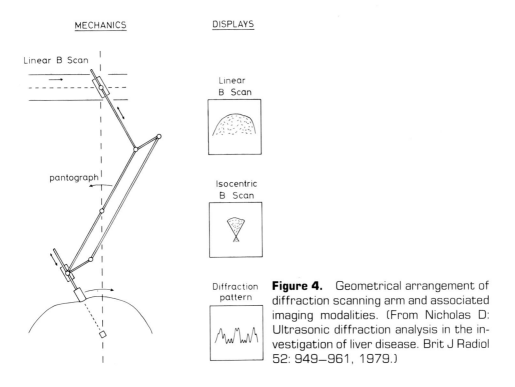

MECHANICS

Linear B Scan

pantograph

DISPLAYS

Linear
B Scan

Isocentric
B Scan

Diffraction
pattern

Figure 4. Geometrical arrangement of diffraction scanning arm and associated imaging modalities. (From Nicholas D: Ultrasonic diffraction analysis in the investigation of liver disease. Brit J Radiol 52: 949–961, 1979.)

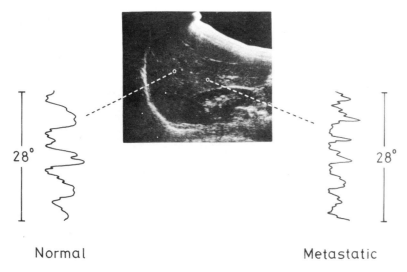

28°

28°

Normal

Metastatic

Figure 5. Liver scan and diffraction patterns from a patient with a focal metastatic deposit: *right*, focal lesion; *left*, normal liver tissue.

31

vestigation of the tissue—a technique that has met with some success in vitro (45) but that is still far from clinical implementation.

TISSUE DYNAMICS

"Real-time" B-scanning has provided a completely new technique for imaging soft tissues and, especially, their motions. Simple imaging techniques now are widely used for monitoring fetal activity, respiration and heart rates and as such are the preferred investigative procedures. In studies of the adult heart (46) time motion scans, the acoustic equivalent of the electrocardiogram, permit a quantitative assessment of both the degree of boundary motion and its direction. Methods based on detection of Doppler frequency shift are also well established and have proved to be of immense value in recording blood flow velocities both in the heart and in major vessels. Doppler also has been used with a fair degree of success in characterizing malignant and benign breast lesions (47). Its full potential as a tissue discriminator has yet to be realized.

Originally, the fluctuation in the speckle representing tissue parenchyma, as visualized with real-time machines, was considered an artifact of the system and, consequently, ignored. Recently, interest in these speckle changes has focused on the possibility that such changes are dictated by bulk acoustic properties of the tissue, such as rigidity or compressibility (41). In the attempt to quantitatively monitor intensity changes in the spatial location of echoes, two techniques have been adopted.

I (48) have conducted a pilot study in which the diffraction technique (described in the previous section) was used to monitor changes in backscattered

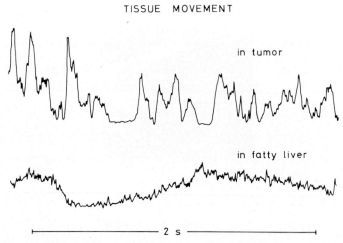

TISSUE   MOVEMENT

in tumor

in fatty liver

2 s

Figure 6.   In vivo diffraction pattern changes as a function of time, performed at 2.5 MHz with a gate length of 10 μs. *Upper trace*: movements within a liver secondary metastasis; *lower trace*: movements within an enlarged liver with fatty infiltration. (From Nicholas D: The analysis of soft tissue movements. In Thijssen JM (ed): Ultrasonic Tissue Characterization. Brussels, Staflen, 1981, pp 281–285.)

intensity as a function of time. Inasmuch as the diffraction technique has been described elsewhere (40, 43) it is sufficient to note that by time-gating the A-scan pertaining to a selected direction a small tissue volume (typically 30 mm^3) can be investigated in reference to its backscattering characteristics. Any changes in tissue volume (with different scatterers entering and/or leaving the time-gate) will result in changes in the interference effects recorded. Although such measurements are unable to provide information on the degree of movement, they are extremely sensitive to small-scale local motions. Figure 6 illustrates diffraction-movement patterns for two liver conditions. The upper trace represents movements within a degenerating secondary liver metastasis. The lower trace is from a grossly enlarged liver with fatty infiltration. Changes in the diffraction information can occur very rapidly in comparison with the heart cycle and may be related to the general "pliability" of the tissues concerned.

Dickinson and Hill (49) monitor consecutive A-scans originating from a predetermined line scan as a function of time, which makes it possible to correlate identical time regions of the A-scans to yield a quantitative description of tissue motions. Both these approaches are in their infancy, yet they indicate that this hitherto neglected aspect of ultrasonic diagnosis may well prove to be of paramount importance in differentiating pathological conditions.

OTHER TECHNIQUES

It is worthwhile to mention techniques which, although different from conventional pulse-echo technology, provide a useful method for in vivo tissue characterization.

Ultrasonic computer-assisted tomography (50) is of considerable interest for determining velocity, attenuation and (possibly) scattering. The presentation of the data as a two-dimensional map or image is acceptable to clinicians for visual assessment and as a quantitative description of the acoustic properties associated with small tissue volumes. Like x-ray computer-assisted tomography, ultrasonic attenuation and velocity maps are based on through transmission of a radiated beam. With ultrasound this is only practicable for superficial organs, of which the breast is the principal example. At present, the velocity maps seem to be the most interesting, and the early in vivo results seem promising, in particular those of Glover (51). He found that abnormally high sound velocity is associated with malignant tissue within the female breast.

The general inability to obtain through transmission of ultrasound in other regions of the human body has lead to consideration of reconstruction techniques based on backscattered data. A preliminary study by Duck and Hill (52) indicated that backscatter maps could be achieved in vitro, though the precise quantitative nature of the data remains open to question.

Other imaging modalities, such as holography (53) and the transmission camera of Green (54) have been used in vivo and do provide useful diagnostic information. However, they are not generally considered for tissue characterization purposes and will not be discussed here.

CONCLUSION

In this brief review, I have attempted to stress techniques which currently complement conventional ultrasound diagnosis. The general goal of these techniques is to quantify data pertaining to the interaction of ultrasound with tissue and to separate out factors relating to specific properties of the tissue volume examined. The described techniques all utilize pulse-echo equipment where conventional B-scan imaging is merely one of several methods available for interpreting the acoustic information.

The possible applications and adaptations of ultrasonic tissue characterization techniques are numerous, and a full appreciation of their diagnostic worth has still to be achieved. The indications for the future are promising, and hopefully, the integration of such techniques into standard diagnostic practice will be forthcoming.

REFERENCES

1. White DN (ed): Recent Advances in Ultrasound in Biomedicine, Vol 1. Forest Grove, Oregon, Research Studies Press, 1977.
2. Hill CR: Tissue Characterization. In Kurjak A (ed): Progress in Medical Ultrasound, Vol 1. Amsterdam, Excerpta Medica, 1980, pp 11–18.
3. Thijssen JM (ed): Ultrasonic Tissue Characterization. Brussels, Stafleu, 1980.
4. Chivers RC: Tissue characterization. Ultrasound Med Biol 7: 1–20, 1981.
5. Wild JJ, Reid JM: Further pilot echographic studies on the histological structures of tumours of the living intact human breast. Am J Path 28: 839–861, 1952.
6. Pohlmann R: Über die Absorption des Ultraschalls im menschlichen Geweben und ihre Abhängigkeit von der Frequenz. Phys Zeit 40: 159–161, 1939.
7. Kossoff G: Measurements using ultrasonic techniques. Proc Roy Soc Med 67: 135–140, 1974.
8. Kossoff G, Garrett WJ, Carpenter DA, et al: Principles and classifications of soft tissues by grey-scale echography. Ultrasound Med Biol 2: 89–106, 1976.
9. Taylor KJW: The principles underlying the classification of soft tissues imaged by reflection techniques with non-linear amplifications (grey-scale). In White DN (ed): Recent Advances in Ultrasound in Biomedicine, Vol 1. Forest Grove, Oregon, Research Studies Press, 1977, pp 157–171.
10. Ossoinig KC: Quantitative echography—the basis of tissue differentiation. J Clin Ultrasound 2: 33–46, 1974.
11. Buschmann W: Tumours of the eye and orbit. In Hill CR, McCready VR, Cosgrove DO (Eds.): Ultrasound in Tumour Diagnosis. Tunbridge Wells, Pitman Medical, 1978, pp 48–66.
12. Mountford RA, Wells PNT: Ultrasonic liver scanning: the quantitative analysis of the normal A-scan. Phys Med Biol 17: 14–25, 1972.
13. Mountford RA, Wells PNT: Ultrasonic liver scanning: the A-scan in the normal and cirrhotic liver. Phys Med Biol 17: 261–269, 1972.
14. Joseph AEA, Dewbury KC, McGuire PG: Ultrasound in the detection of chronic liver disease. Br J Radiol 52: 184–188, 1979.

15. Dewbury KC, Clark B: The accuracy of ultrasound in the detection of cirrhosis of the liver. Br J Radiol 52: 945–948, 1979.

16. Lerski RA, Barnett E, Morley P, et al: Computer analysis of ultrasonic signals in diffuse liver disease. Ultrasound Med Biol 5: 341–250, 1979.

17. Linzer M (Ed): Ultrasonic Tissue Characterization I. NBS Special Publication 453. Washington, U.S. Dept. of Commerce, 1976.

18. Hill CR, Chivers RC, Huggins RW, et al: Scattering of ultrasound by human tissue. In Fry FJ (Ed): Ultrasound: Its Applications in Medicine and Biology. Amsterdam, Elsevier, 1978, pp 441–493.

19. Goss SA, Johnson RL, Dunn F: Comprehensive compilation of empirical ultrasonic properties of mammalian tissues. J Acoust Soc Am 64: 423–457, 1978.

20. Kuc R: Clinical application of an ultrasound attenuation coefficient estimation technique for liver pathology characterization. IEEE Trans Biomed Eng 27: 312–319, 1980.

21. Lizzi FL, St. Louis L, Coleman DJ: Applications of spectral analysis in medical ultrasonography. Ultrasonics 14: 77–80, 1976.

22. Lizzi FL, Coleman DJ: Ultrasonic spectrum analysis in ophthalmology: In White DN (ed): Recent Advances in Ultrasound in Biomedicine, Vol 1. Forest Grove, Oregon, Research Studies Press, 1977, pp 117–129.

23. Nicholas D: The application of acoustic scattering parameters to the characterization of human soft tissues. Proceedings of the IEEE Ultrasonics Symposium. New York, IEEE, 1976, pp 64–69.

24. Shung KK, Reid JM: Ultrasonic scattering from tissues. Proceedings of the IEEE Ultrasonics Symposium. New York, IEEE, 1977, pp 230–233.

25. Freese M, Lyons EA: Ultrasonic backscatter from human liver tissue: its dependence on frequency and protein/lipid composition. J Clin Ultrasound 5: 307–312, 1977.

26. Nicholas D: Evaluation of backscattering coefficient for excised human tissues: results, interpretation and associated measurements. Ultrasound Med Biol 8: 17–28, 1982.

27. Lizzi FL, Laviola MA, Coleman DJ: Tissue signature characterization utilising frequency domain characterization. Proceedings of the IEEE Ultrasonics Symposium. New York, IEEE, 1976, pp 714–719.

28. Sommer FG, Joynt LF, Carroll BA, et al: Ultrasonic characterization of abdominal tissues via digital analysis of backscattered waveforms. Radiology 141: 811–817, 1982.

29. Sommer FG, Joynt LF, Hayes DL, et al: Stochastic frequency-domain tissue characterization: application to human spleens *in vivo*. Ultrasonics 20: 82–86, 1982.

30. Jones JP: Impediography: a new ultrasonic technique for diagnostic medicine. In White DN (ed): Ultrasound in Medicine, Vol 1. New York, Plenum Press, 1975, pp 489–497.

31. Kak AC, Fry FJ, Jones JP: Acoustic impedance profiling. In Fry FJ (Ed): Ultrasound: Its Applications in Medicine and Biology. Amsterdam, Elsevier, 1978, pp 495–537.

32. Jones JP: *In vivo* characterization of several lesions in the eye using ultrasonic impediography. In Metherell AF (Ed): Acoustical Imaging, Vol 8, New York, Plenum Press, 1980, pp 539–546.

33. Robinson DE, Kossoff G: Line mode echogram data acquisition and computer re-

construction techniques. In Kurjak A (Ed): Recent Advances in Ultrasound Diagnosis 2. Amsterdam, Excerpta Medica, 1979, pp 44–47.

34. Nicholas D, Barrett A, Chu JMG, et al: Computer analysis of grey-scale tomograms. In Metherell AF (Ed): Acoustical Imaging, Vol 8. New York, Plenum Press, 1980, pp 731–744.

35. Nicholas D: Pre- and post-processing of images held on temporary storage devices. In Hill CR, Kratochwil A (Eds): Medical Ultrasonic Images: Formation, Display, Recording and Perception. Amsterdam, Excerpta Medica, 1981, pp 61–68.

36. Waag RC, Lee PPK, Gramiak R: Digital processing to enhance features of ultrasonic images. Proceedings of the IEEE Computer Society Conference on Patter Recognition and Image Processing. New York, IEEE, 1978, pp 1–7.

37. Wessells G, Seelen W, Scheiding U: The application of pattern recognition in ultrasonic sectional pictures of the prostate (B-mode analysis). In Thijssen JM (Ed): Ultrasonic Tissue Characterization. Brussels, Staflen, 1981, pp 273–280.

38. Lorenz WJ, Bihl H, van Kaick G, Lorenz A, et al: Methods of image analysis and enhancement. In Hill CR, Kratochwil A (Eds): Medical Ultrasonic Images: Formation, Display, Recording and Perception. Amsterdam, Excerpta Medica, 1981, pp 69–76.

39. Nicholas D, Bamber M, Bossi C, et al: Quantitative image analysis for diffuse liver disease. Ultrasonic Imaging 3: 186, 1981.

40. Nicholas D, Hill CR: Acoustic Bragg diffraction from human tissues. Nature 257: 305–306, 1975.

41. Nicholas D: Orientation and frequency dependence of backscattered energy and its clinical application. In White DN (Ed): Recent Advances in Ultrasound in Biomedicine, Vol 1, Forest Grove, Oregon, Research Studies Press, 1977, pp 29–54.

42. Huggins RW, Phelps J: Bragg diffraction scanner for ultrasonic tissue characterization *in vivo*. Ultrasound Med Biol 2: 271–277, 1976.

43. Nicholas D: Ultrasonic diffraction analysis in the investigation of liver disease. Br J Radiol 52: 949–961, 1979.

44. Merton J, Nicholas D, Hill CR, et al: Ultrasonic diffraction scanning of the thyroid. Ultrasound Med Biol 8: 145–153, 1982.

45. Nicholas AW, Nicholas D: The analysis of three-dimensional tissue structures using ultrasound diffraction patterns. Phys Med Biol 25: 759, 1980.

46. Vogel JA, Bastiaans OL, Bom K et al: M-mode computations and two-dimensional image reconstruction. In Kurjak A (Ed): Recent Advances in Ultrasound Diagnosis 2. Amsterdam, Excerpta Medica, 1979, pp 48–54.

47. Wells PNT, Halliwell M, Skidmore R, et al: Tumour detection by ultrasonic Doppler blood flow signals. Ultrasonics 15: 231–232, 1977.

48. Nicholas D: The analysis of soft tissue movements. In Thijssen JM (Ed): Ultrasonic Tissue Characterization. Brussels, Staflen, 1981, pp 281–285.

49. Dickinson RJ, Hill CR: Measurement of soft tissue motion using correlation between A-scans. Ultrasound Med Biol 8: 263–271.

50. Greenleaf JF, Johnson SA, Lee SL, et al: Algebraic reconstruction of spatial distributions of acoustic absorption within tissue from their two-dimensional acoustic projections. In Green PS (Ed): Acoustic Holography, Vol 5. New York, Plenum Press, 1974, pp 589–599.

51. Glover GH: Computerized time-of-flight ultrasonic tomography for breast examination. Ultrasound Med Biol 3: 117–128, 1977.

52. Duck FA, Hill CR: Acoustic attenuation reconstruction from backscattered ultrasound. In Raviv J, Greenleaf JF, Hermen GT (Eds): Computer Aided Tomography and Ultrasonics in Medicine. Amsterdam, North Holland Publishing Company, 1979, pp 137–149.

53. Chivers RC: Acoustical holography. In White DN (Ed): Recent Advances in Ultrasound in Biomedicine, Vol 1. Forest Grove, Oregon, Research Studies Press, 1977, pp 217–251.

54. Green PS, Saefer LF, Jones ED, et al: A new high performance ultrasonic camera system. In Green PS (Ed): Acoustical Holography, Vol 5. New York, Plenum Press, 1974, pp 493–507.

4

USE OF PRESCAN AND POSTSCAN SIGNAL PROCESSING IN ULTRASONIC CANCER DIAGNOSIS

Morimichi Fukuda

Ultrasound imaging is a very useful clinical tool primarily because it displays echo position and amplitude to produce static as well as moving cross-sectional images of the living human body (1–3).

The introduction of grey scale signal processing with improved transducer design and use of digital scan converters have radically changed the concept of ultrasonography. Grey scale ultrasound is used extensively in a variety of clinical situations because of its simplicity and accuracy and because it does not present the various biomedical hazards that often accompany x-ray diagnosis and nuclear medicine.

It has been found that considerable experience is necessary if one is to diagnose malignant tumors by sonography. In the ultrasonic examination of the liver, for example, there are differences in the way in which the echo patterns of primary and metastatic carcinoma have been described (4–11). These discrepancies seem to have arisen for various reasons, e.g., the use of different instruments, differences in the populations examined, a lack of quantitative data, and the lower resolution of sonograms.

Diagnostic difficulties are gradually being overcome by improved instruments that use focused transducers with increased sensitivity, signal processing for image enhancement (12, 13), improved real-time techniques (12–15), signal amplification and grey scale technology (4, 16–18).

Advances also are being made in the area of ultrasonic tissue characterization. Studies are focusing on such features as wave velocity, attenuation and reflection characteristics. Several other factors associated with image quality and character, including the roughness of mass contours, shadowing, internal echo amplitude and the location of masses are also under investigation. Tissue characterization studies have been summarized in a series of symposia sponsored by the National Bureau of Standards of the United States held over the last 5 years. A review of this subject may be found in Chapters 1–3 of this book.

In the area of ultrasonic image pattern characteristics, a number of studies have been reported. Kobayashi et al (19, 20) have correlated echo patterns with histopathological findings. They found that benign tumors usually display a smoothly outlined mass filled with tiny, uniform echoes, the posterior echoes showing slight attenuation or enhancement, depending upon the size and attenuating properties of the tumor parenchyma. Malignant tumors, on the other hand, showed much more complex echo patterns. The margin of the tumor invariably exhibited irregular contours, with internal echoes also showing considerable heterogeneity both in size and echo intensity and posterior echoes often disappearing due to the increased attenuation caused by the higher collagen content of the tumor tissues, especially in the case of scirrhous-type carcinoma of the breast.

Also, a number of workers are involved in studies of quantitative aspects of tumor tissues. Fry and her colleagues (21), employing the fast Fourier transform method, have shown that a significant attenuation of sonic waves occurs in cancer tissue of the breast. Entirely different approaches to the elucidation of tissue changes in malignancies by ultrasound have been reported by Hill and Nicholas (cf. Chapter 3).

Computerized ultrasonic tomography using through-transmission projection to obtain data on attenuation of or on changes in ultrasonic propagation speed and reconstruction of two-dimensional images has achieved only limited success due to the difficulties involved in the mathematical computation of results (22–24).

Wells et al (25) have emphasized the employment of Doppler-shift techniques as a method for tissue classification of breast carcinoma based upon changes in the blood flow possibly caused by neovascularization of malignant neoplastic changes.

In spite of these efforts aimed at achieving early detection of the malignant transformation, practical applications of the studies remain limited.

The following paragraphs summarize some of our work concerning the characterization of hepatic malignancies (5, 12, 14).

SENSITIVITY-GRADED ULTRASONOGRAPHY

Sensitivity-graded ultrasonography was first introduced by Kikuchi in 1968 (26) to quantitatively assess the echo signals arising from malignant tumors and normal tissues. The method is rather complicated, the principle being the comparison of echo intensities of normal and cancerous tissues by means of a margin test. Clinically, the method is cumbersome and the extensive ultrasonic equipment necessary makes the original method impractical. Kikuchi has since advocated a simplified version of the method, designated "sensitivity-graded tomography pairs," for evaluation of the echogenicity of lesions.

The objective of this simplified version is to record several scans of the same section of a suspected organ using increments of system sensitivity, preferably in 3- or 6-dB steps. As the sensitivity is stepped up or down, some significant echoes will appear or disappear. One of the physiological echoes arising from normal tissue located at the same depth from the scanning transducer is used as the reference sensitivity (5, 26). The echo level of the lesion is determined by comparison of the echogenicity of the target with the reference sensitivity, the difference being expressed as the sensitivity value in decibels. A similar technique has been used by Kobayashi et al (19) for classification of the echo patterns of breast carcinoma and by me for liver tumors (5).

This method is semiquantitative and is more accurate for the description of echo intensities of tumors than the simple visual estimate of a single grey scale echogram recorded at a wide dynamic range setting. As recently reported by Taylor (27), evaluation of echogenicity from a single grey scale echogram can yield an erroneous interpretation of the echogenicity of a lesion because transducers operating at different frequencies and focused differently generally are used to obtain better resolution. Although resolution may be improved, the fidelity of system sensitivity with regard to the echo intensity of the lesion may be seriously impaired, especially if the lesion is located far from the focused area after maximal time-gain compensation settings. Similar problems have been pointed out by Jaffe and Harris (28). Digitization as performed by modern ultrasonic equipment with digital scan converters produce numerical-intensity values that sometimes have little meaning because they have been modified by a number of factors, such as the use of different transducers, gain settings and variable time-gain compensation.

Table 1 shows my (5) preliminary classification of primary hepatocellular carcinoma of the liver based upon the technique described above. Although the number of cases studied was limited, this was the first report to include the concept of echo levels in the diagnostic evaluation of tumor tissue characteristics.

S-SHAPED AMPLIFICATION OF ECHO SIGNALS FOR B-MODE PRESENTATION

Grey scale echography brought about registration of echoes on an expanded dynamic range without saturation of specular echoes. Nevertheless, in certain cases of hepatocellular carcinoma, as well as in some metastatic tumors of the liver, differences in tissue contrast are so small that optical differentiation of

TABLE 1. Classification of Echo Patterns of Primary Hepatoma (5)

Type 1. *Circumscribed Nodular Pattern*
A round tumor mass is surrounded by a sonoluscent halo, which becomes prominent on sequential attenuation. The levels and distribution of echoes of the mass closely resemble those of normal parenchyma, the maximum echo difference being only 6–9 dB higher than normal liver tissue.

Type 2. *Nodular Pattern with Irregular Contours*
The surrounding halo is less prominent and the contours of the tumor mass rather irregular; the echo levels of the tumor frequently exceed by 12 dB or more those of normal parenchyma.

Type 3. *Diffuse, Irregular Spotted Pattern with Lowered Echo Levels*
The echo levels of the mass are 6 dB or more lower than those of normal tissue and the tumor mass is sharply outlined against the normal tissue.

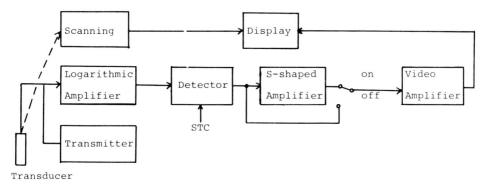

Figure 1. Block diagram of S-shaped amplification apparatus for B-mode presentation.

tumor tissues from the surrounding tissue is difficult. Tumors of this nature can be missed unless one looks at gross morphological alterations such as the hump sign, the edge sign or marked displacement of the intracellular vasculatures.

To overcome these difficulties inherent in grey scale portrayal of echo signals, various prescan processing schemes, such as changes in assignment of grey levels on the basis of amplitude of echo (13), line-mode echogram data acquisition and computer reconstruction techniques (29) and S-shaped amplification of echo signals (30, 31) have been employed. The last method, first reported by Patel and Ossoinig (30), who used S-shaped amplification of echo signals for A-mode presentation of intraocular tumors, was found to be applicable to the B-mode presentation and assessment of hepatic neoplasms (12).

As is shown in Figure 1, echo signals received by the transducer were fed to a logarithmic amplifier and then led to a detector where the time-gain compensation functions regulated the final echo amplitude before the signal was amplified to the S-shaped amplifier. The echoes can be fed either directly to a videoamplifier (original grey scale mode) or through the S-shaped amplifier by an on-off switch in the circuit. The resulting signal was fed to the display unit to produce the B-mode image via a scan converter. The amplification characteristics were manually controlled by manipulating 17 sliding switches on the front panel of the amplifier (Figure 2). The abscissa and ordinate indicate the input dynamic range from the logarithmic amplifier and the resulting intensity of the output of the S-shaped amplifier unit, respectively. Accordingly, various amplification curves could be generated. It soon became apparent, however, that the most important part of the curve, especially for the effective visualization of intrahepatic tumors, was the steepness of the lower end, i.e., the method for extending the low-level echo display.

Figures 3 and 4 present a typical example of the effect of S-shaped amplification. As is shown in Figure 4, recording a sonogram at a single gain setting often results in an unsatisfactory image. When the gain settings of the equipment were increased in a stepwise fashion, it was possible to progressively elucidate fine details of the malignant tumors.

Figure 5 shows two sonograms of the liver of a patient with suspected ad-

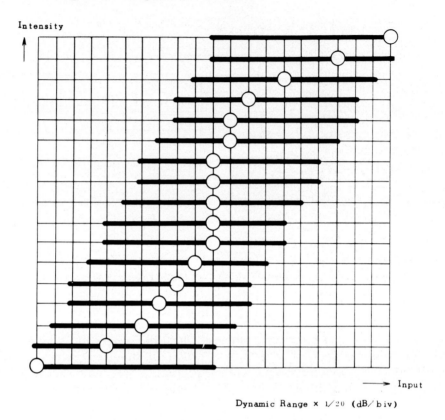

Figure 2.   Program of transfer characteristic used for S-shaped amplification of echo signals.

vanced liver cirrhosis recorded by intercostal scanning with the patient in the left decubital position. The grey scale image without signal processing failed to show any discrete masses in the liver, except for some fine echo spots distributed throughout the liver. Ascitic fluid in the peritoneal cavity also was seen. The S-shaped amplification was accompanied by successive increases in overall gain settings. The peculiar echo pattern shown in Figure 5 demonstrates echogenic masses distributed over the entire liver lobe and leaving the hypoechoic rim in the periphery. The patient died of acutely aggravated cachexia 3 weeks after sonography was performed. Necropsy revealed advanced hepatocellular carcinoma accompanied by cirrhosis of the liver. The surface of the liver, cut in the same plane as the echogram, (Figure 5, bottom) shows hepatomas coinciding exactly with those portrayed in the echogram. Histopathological examination disclosed well-advanced annular cirrhosis of the liver and moderately differentiated hepatocellular carcinoma superimposed on the preexisting cirrhotic liver tissue.

Figure 6 shows another set of echograms typical of hepatocellular carcinoma recorded using the same amplification curve. Here, with the gain setting increasing from 75 to 85 dB, a large tumor mass occupying the central portion

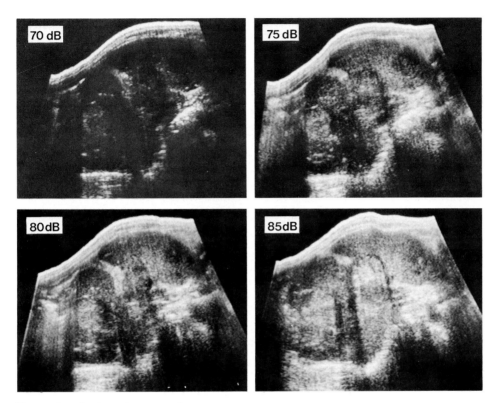

Figure 3. Series of grey scale sonograms of primary hepatocellular carcinoma (right subcostal scan) recorded at gain settings of 70, 75, 80 and 85 dB.

of the liver is clearly distinguishable from the noncancerous portion of the liver. The latter was found to be more echogenic in the nonprocessed grey scale echogram. The margin of the tumor was also obscured, as the figure illustrates. Although manual contact-compound scanning was used to record these echograms, the resolution was adequate for tissue differentiation.

In patients with metastatic carcinoma of the liver, image processing is not required, because the echogenicity of the lesion is distinctly different. However, S-shaped amplification is often useful when more detailed analysis of echogenic and hypoechoic tumors is required.

Figure 7 shows a series of echograms from a patient with colonic carcinoma metastasized to the liver. Contact-compound scanning along the right subcostal margin disclosed two large masses with slightly increased echo levels. The increase in gain disclosed marked heterogeneity of the internal structure of the tumor nodules, as is evident from the echograms. On-off mode settings showed that the difference between echogenic and less echogenic portions of the liver was 15 dB. Figure 8 shows echograms from another patient suffering gastric scirrhous carcinoma metastasized to the liver. The original and processed echograms are similar to those presented in Figure 7. The histological

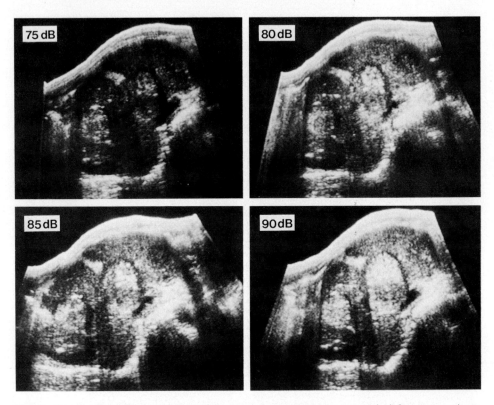

Figure 4. Series of preprocessed grey scale sonograms recorded from a patient with primary hepatocellular carcinoma at gain settings of 75, 80, 85 and 90 dB. Tissue contrast is markedly increased after the processing, and the abnormality of the echo level of the hepatoma nodules is clearly demonstrated.

section of the liver prepared after necropsy showed infiltration of the liver by metastasizing adenocarcinoma. The liver was quite heterogeneous, consisting of portions rich in connective tissue, necrotic foci accompanied by bleeding and massive adenocarcinoma infiltration.

Even in hypoechoic nodules, a stepwise increase in gain setting revealed features specific to malignant tissue, such as a mass filled with fine, irregular echo spots and a jagged border.

S-shaped amplification in more than 800 patients with malignant and non-malignant diseases revealed only two cases of advanced liver cirrhosis exhibiting quasimalignant patterns. Absence of malignant tumors in these patients was confirmed by examination with a high-resolution real-time scanner.

POSTSCAN IMAGE PROCESSING

Postprocessing, defined as an alteration of the digitized pixel amplitude codes so as to redistribute the final output of grey levels on the display, is another

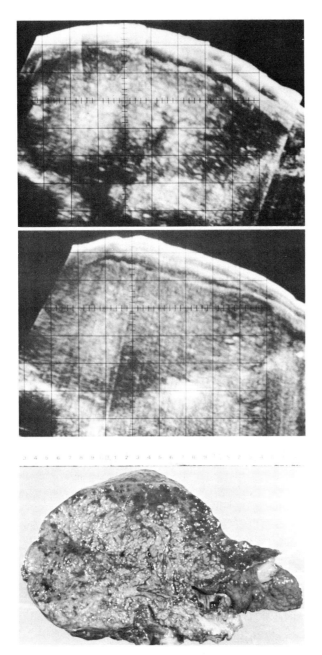

Figure 5. Comparison of B mode images with and without S-shaped amplification from a patient with hepatocellular carcinoma. The top image, recorded with S-shaped amplification, clearly shows higher echo levels from the tumor tissue than the bottom image, recorded without processing. The cut surface of the liver photographed at the time of necropsy is also shown.

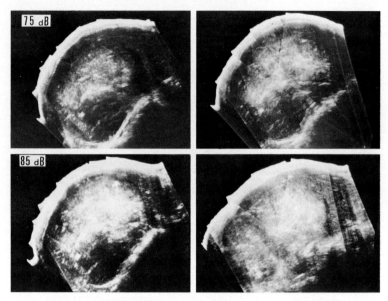

Figure 6. Comparison of B-mode images recorded from a patient suffering hepatocellular carcinoma with and without S-shaped amplification. *Left top and bottom:* S-shaped amplification on; *right top and bottom:* S-shaped amplification off.

important development. The method is similar to preprocessing, except that it is performed after image formation without affecting the original image data, which is stored in the scan converter memory (13, 24, 29, 32).

AMPLITUDE PROCESSING

Original data stored in digitized form can be displayed by the image-processing functions incorporated in some equipment. A linear mode indicates each increment in the coded pixel level, producing an equal step in the displayed brightness, that is, the original grey scale sonogram is displayed on the screen.

To increase optical differentiation, various optional programs, such as "weak echo expand" or "strong echo expand," that is, the mapping of weak or strong echo signals into, for instance, three-quarters of the luminescence variations, have been incorporated into the equipment. Other selections, such as expansion or compression of the "midrange" echoes or thresholding of weaker or higher pixel values to vary the dynamic range of the image, also can be made. Examples of these signal-processing techniques are shown in Figure 9.

Generally, the postprocessing schemes assign a relatively broad range of grey levels to low and midrange echoes, providing, for example, increased contrast display of liver metastases and enhanced contrast between pancreas and liver.

In an attempt to optimize image data processing, I have applied an S-shaped amplification method as was used in the preprocessing experiments just described. On the basis of experience obtained in the preprocessing of B-mode images, I selected three amplification curves and incorporated them into the postprocessing functions (Figure 10). These S-shaped curves were digitized into 6 bits to yield 64 shapes of gray in the display. After the B-mode image was stored by contact compound scanning, four postprocessed images were obtained instantaneously by manipulation of the dial on the front panel of the instrument.

Another important consideration, apart from enhanced tissue contrast, is the delineation or extraction of echographic features characteristic of a malignant lesion. Figure 11 illustrates an original transverse echogram of a slightly swollen pancreatic body and the images processed with three S-curved functions. The image treated by S-curve D, which generates a rather narrow

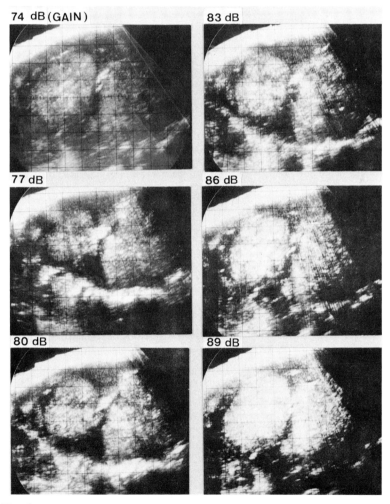

Figure 7. A series of preprocessed sonograms of colon cancer metastasized to the liver at six gain settings.

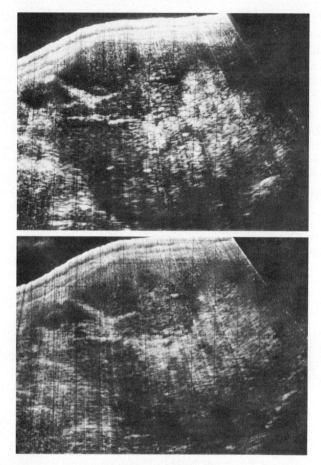

Figure 8. Comparison of B mode images recorded from a patient with gastric carcinoma metastasized to the liver. Preprocessing with S-shaped amplification (*top*) markedly enhanced the tissue contrast of the metastatic nodules.

dynamic range image, clearly shows the irregularity of the contour of the swollen pancreatic body (the zigzag sign), indicating the malignancy of the lesion. The S-curve B treatment showed some spotty abnormal echoes inside the swollen parenchyma of the pancreas. In the course of this study, these two features frequently were very useful, that is, the contour and the abnormality of the internal echo characteristics as revealed by the postprocessing method were frequently used to characterize malignant neoplasms.

Figure 12 demonstrates another such example, in which a transverse echogram of a case of abdominal Hodgkin's disease was processed according to the S-curves present. The original grey scale echogram showed a slight degree of echo saturation, especially of those arising from the swollen lymph node-like structures shown in the middle of the figure. As expected, the individual lymph node contours become more prominent after processing by curve B and C and are slightly too bright after processing by curve D. These results clearly

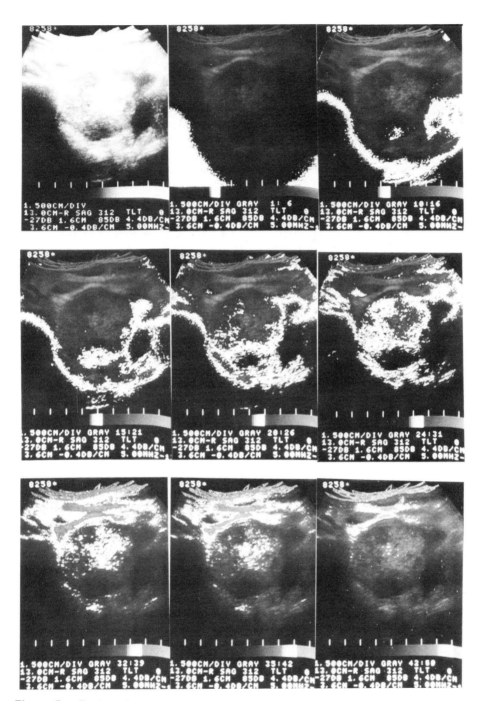

Figure 9. Series of echograms obtained by postprocessing of an image recorded in a digital scan converter. Windowing of the grey scale tomogram at different levels certainly depicts areas of a particular amplitude level, but the original sonogram allows much clear recognition of the tumor mass as a whole.

49

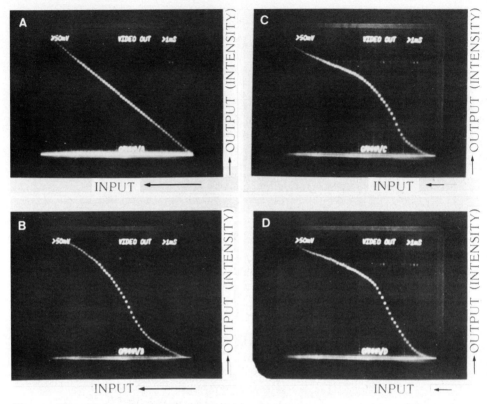

Figure 10. S-shaped amplification curves used in postscan processing (Aloka SSD180BL). Curve A: original logarithmic amplification. Curves B, C and D: respective S-shaped amplification. abscissa: input voltage. ordinate: output (intensity).

indicate that even a seemingly saturated echogram may be processed effectively by S-shaped amplification.

The most important prerequisite of effective image processing is the precise registration of echoes, in terms of both geometry and echogenicity. This registration was difficult with the conventional contact compound scanner. Recent improvement in the design of scanning instruments have made it possible to carry out these requirements without difficulty. Figure 13 shows an echogram delineating malignant lesions in the liver of a 17-year-old boy with hepatomegaly and a positive AFP test obtained with an Aloka SSD 180 BL with a 5 MHz transducer 13 mm in diameter. A transverse tomogram of the upper abdomen disclosed a marked enlargement of the entire liver, which contained a number of slightly echogenic foci suggestive of primary hepatocellular carcinoma. A small echogenic nodule in the right lobe of the liver was enlarged four times using the "read-zoom" mode, and various postprocessing schemes were applied to increase tissue contrast and reveal the contours of the nodule. The contour irregularity and marked heterogeneity in the echogenicity of the nodule shown in the figure strongly suggested a malignant lesion. Echo-guided aspiration cytology later confirmed hepatocellular carcinoma.

It is premature to say that the amplitude postprocessing of B-mode is effec-

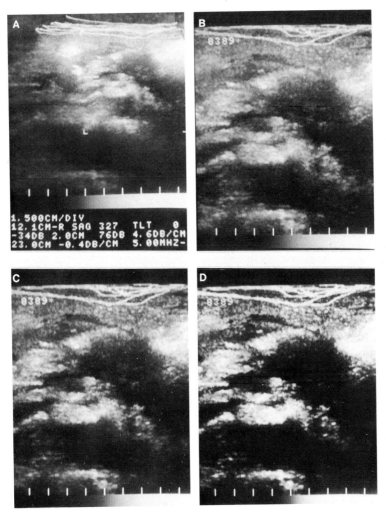

Figure 11. Comparison of sonograms of cancer of the body of the pancreas before and after postprocessing according to the programs shown in Figure 10. A portion of the transverse tomogram as marked in the figure was twofold by "read zoom" and postprocessed. The sonogram treated by curve D clearly exhibits contour irregularity, whereas the sonogram treated by curve B shows ill-defined abnormal echo spots in the tumor parenchyma.

tive in tumor differential diagnosis. Nevertheless, the experience gained so far supports and justifies the use of this technique to enhance the optical assessment of tumor characteristics.

STATISTICAL POSTPROCESSING

The image stored in a digital scan converter may be accessed for various computations by a computer. The data may be processed to produce smoothed or

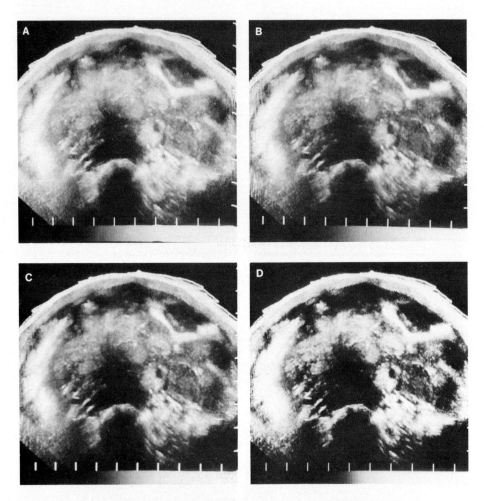

Figure 12. Comparison of sonograms of abdominal Hodgkin's disease. The transverse tomogram of the lower abdomen shows numerous lymph node-like structures, which become much more apparent after treatment by curves B–D.

filtered images. It is also possible to count the number of pixels of each amplitude in the image and construct an amplitude-histogram demonstrating the relative number of echoes of each strength in a particular area in the image. Amplitude histogram analysis has been used (33) successfully to differentiate between pancreatic parenchymal tissues of normal patients and those suffering mucoviscidosis. There are few other reports on the use of statistical data in tissue discrimination.

High-resolution real-time scanners equipped with either a linear-array or an annular-array transducer combined with a dynamic focusing method undoubtedly also will yield important diagnostic clues based on the recognition of changes in tissue texture caused by malignant transformation and on the visualization of distortion of normal vasculatures by infiltrating cancer tissues.

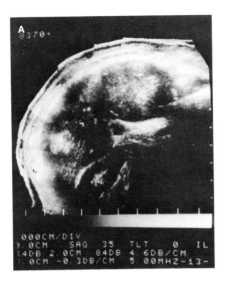

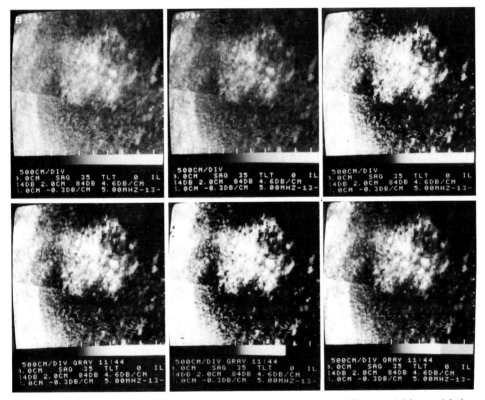

Figure 13. (*A*) A grey scale tomogram recorded from a 17-year-old boy with hepatocellular carcinoma. (*B*) A portion of the sonogram recorded in the digital scan converter was enlarged by the "read-zoom" mode and postprocessed by different settings. A jagged contour and marked heterogeneity of the internal echo amplitude are apparent.

ACKNOWLEDGMENT

This work was supported in part by Grant-in-Aid for Cancer Research 57-1 from the Ministry of Health and Welfare of Japan.

REFERENCES

1. Wells PNT: Biomedical Ultrasonics. London, Academic Press, 1977.
2. Wild JJ: The use of ultrasonic pulses for the measurement of biological tissues and the determination of tissue density changes. Surgery 27: 183–188, 1950.
3. Wild JJ: The use of pulse-echo ultrasound for early tumor detection: history and prospects. In Hill CR, et al (eds): Ultrasound in Tumour Diagnosis. Tunbridge Wells, Pitman Medical, 1978, pp 1–26.
4. Cosgrove DO: Evaluation of liver tumours. In Hill CR (ed): Ultrasound in Tumour Diagnosis. Tunbridge Wells, Pitman Medical, 1978, pp 104–127.
5. Fukuda M: Evaluation of sensitivity graded ultrasonotomography in diagnosis of malignant tumors of upper abdominal organs. In White DN, Brown R (eds): Ultrasound in Medicine, Vol 3A. New York, Plenum Press, 1977, pp 303–314.
6. Green B, Bree RL, Goldstein HM, et al: Gray scale ultrasound evaluation of hepatic neoplasms: patterns and correlations. Radiology 124: 203–208, 1977.
7. Kossoff G: Classification of soft tissues by grey scale echography. In White DN, Brown R (eds): Ultrasound in Medicine, Vol 3B. New York, Plenum Press, 1977, pp 1869–1874.
8. Scheible W, Gosink BB, Leopold GR: Gray scale echographic patterns of hepatic metastatic disease. Am J Roentgenol Radium Ther Nucl Med 129: 983–987, 1977.
9. Taylor KJW, Carpenter DA, McCready VK: Grey scale echography in the diagnosis of intrahepatic diseases. J Clin Ultrasound 1: 284–287, 1973.
10. Viscomi GN, Gonzalez R, Taylor KJW: Histopathological correlation of ultrasonic appearance of liver metastasis. Proceedings 24th Annual Meeting of American Institute of Ultrasound in Medicine, AIUM, Montreal, 1979, p 19.
11. Weill FS: Ultrasonography of Digestive Diseases. St. Louis, The CV Mosby Co, 1978.
12. Fukuda M: Ultrasonic tissue characterization of hepatic and pancreatic malignancies by means of various pulse-echo ultrasound. In Wagai T, Omoto R (eds): Ultrasound in Medicine and Biology. International Congress Series 505. Amsterdam, Excerpta Medica, 1980, pp 151–158.
13. Sommer FG, Rauschkolb TN, Taylor KJW: Enhancement of tissue contrast using currently available pre- and postscan processing. Proceedings 24th Annual Meeting of American Institute of Ultrasound in Medicine, AIUM, Montreal, 1979, p 34.
14. Fukuda M, Uchida R: Ultrasonic Diagnosis of Liver, Bile Duct and Pancreatic Diseases. Tokyo, Kanehara Publishers, 1979.
15. Cosgrove DO, Chu JMG, McCready VR, et al: Clinical trials on a new real-time abdominal scanner. In White DN, Lyons EA (eds): Ultrasound in Medicine, Vol 4. New York, Plenum Press, 1978, pp 81–90.
16. Kossoff G: Improved techniques in ultrasonic cross-sectional echography. Ultrasonics 10: 221, 1972.

17. Kossoff G, Garrett WJ, Carpenter DA, et al: Principles and classification of soft tissues by grey scale echography. Ultrasound Med Biol 2: 89–105, 1976.

18. Taylor KJW, Carpenter DA, Hill CR, et al: Gray scale ultrasound imaging: the anatomy and pathology of the liver. Radiology 119: 415–423, 1976.

19. Kobayashi T, Takatani O, Hattori N, et al: Differential diagnosis of breast tumors: the sensitivity graded method of ultrasonic tomography and clinical evaluation of its diagnostic accuracy. Cancer 33: 940–951, 1974.

20. Kobayashi T: Correlation of ultrasonic attenuation with connective tissue content in breast cancers. In Linzer M (ed): Ultrasonic Tissue Characterization II. National Bureau of Standards, Special Publication 525, 1979, pp 93–99.

21. Fry EK, Sanghvi NT, Fry FJ: Frequency dependent attenuation of malignant breast tumors studied by the fast Fourier transform technique. In Linzer M (ed): Ultrasonic Tissue Characterization II. National Bureau of Standards, Special Publication 525, 1979, pp 85–91.

22. Carson PL, Oughton TV, Hendee WR: Ultrasonic transaxial tomography by reconstruction. In White DN, Barns R (eds): Ultrasound in Medicine, Vol 2. New York, Plenum Press, 1976, p 341–350.

23. Glover GH, Sharp JC: Reconstruction of ultrasound propagation speed distribution in soft tissue: time of flight tomography. IEEE Trans Sonics Ultrasonics. SU-24: 229–234, 1977.

24. Linzer M, Parks JI, Norton SJ, et al: A comprehensive ultrasonic tissue analysis system. In Linzer M (ed): Ultrasonic Tissue Characterization II. National Bureau of Standards. Special Publication 525, 1979, pp 255–259.

25. Wells PNT, Halliwell M, Skidmore R, et al: Tumour detection by ultrasonic Doppler blood flow signals. Ultrasonics 15: 231–232, 1977.

26. Kikuchi Y: Way to quantitative examination in ultrasonic diagnosis. Med Ultrasonics 6: 1–8, 1968.

27. Taylor KJB: Letter to the editor. J Clin Ultrasound 7: 339, 1980.

28. Jaffe CC, Harris DJ: Physical factors influencing numerical echo-amplitude data extracted from B-scan ultrasound images. J Clin Ultrasound 8: 327–333, 1980.

29. Robinson DE, Kossoff G: Computor processing of line mode echogram data. In Wagai T, Omoto R (eds): Ultrasound in Medicine and Biology. International Congress Series 505. Amsterdam, Excerpta Medica, 1980, pp 11–16.

30. Patel JH, Ossoinig KC: A-scan instrumentation for acoustic tissue differentiation. I. Signal processing in the 7200 MA unit of Kretztechnik. In White DN, Brown R (eds): Ultrasound in Medicine, Vol 3B. New York, Plenum Press, 1977, pp 1939–1948.

31. Ossoinig KC, Patel JH: A-scan instrumentation for acoustic tissue differentiation. II. Clinical significance of various technical parameters of the 7200 MA unit of Kretztechnik. In White DN, Brown R (eds): Ultrasound in Medicine, Vol 38. New York, Plenum Press, 1977, 1949–1954.

32. Maginess MG: Signal processing, image storage, and display. In Wells PNT, Ziskin MC (eds): New Techniques and Instrumentation in Ultrasonography. New York, Churchill Livingstone, 1980, pp 40–68.

II

Ultrasonic Diagnosis of Malignant Tumors

5

ULTRASONIC DIFFERENTIAL DIAGNOSIS OF TUMORS IN OPHTHALMOLOGY

Sadanao Tane

Ultrasonography produces sharp images of soft tissues; it is indispensable in identifying intraocular disorders in eyes with opaque media and in diagnosing intraorbital disorders occurring during exophthalmos. In the diagnosis of ocular tumors, ultrasonography is useful in the identification of the site, shape, size, characteristics (inside echo), etc., of intraocular and intraorbital tumors. A more accurate diagnosis can be made by combining ultrasonography with computerized tomography (CT), which is valuable in determining the site of the lesion, with angiography, which demonstrates the condition of blood flow and metabolism, and with other imaging methods, such as thermography and scintigraphy.

In this chapter I will discuss the characteristics of the echo patterns of various ocular tumors and detail criteria for their differential diagnosis. Some of the important diagnostic criteria are as follows:

1) A tumor in the bulb is visualized as an increase in echogenicity and a tumor in the orbit as a decrease in echogenicity.
2) Many serial scans of the bulb and orbit should be made.
3) The diagnosis should be made only after the findings of routine ophthalmic examination, simple x-ray examinations, CT, radioisotope scintigraphy and thermography, have been evaluated.
4) A premature diagnosis from findings obtained from a single examination should be avoided, and the tumor should be watched for changes and growth.
5) Presence of acoustic vacuoles, choroidal excavations and acoustic shadows in intraocular tumors should be watched for. Such findings are often found in malignant tumors but rarely seen in benign tumors or hemorrhagic changes.

6) In quantitative ultrasonography, the ultrasonic attenuation of the malignant tumor is small.

7) Special attention should be paid to marginal echos and sound transmissions when evaluating tumor echos.

CLASSIFICATION OF EXAMINATION METHODS OF OPHTHALMIC DIAGNOSTIC ULTRASONIC EQUIPMENT

For diagnostic accuracy, precise diagnostic ultrasonic equipment is required. Ultrasonic equipment used in ophthalmology today can be divided into four groups by the way contact is made with the eye.

1) Contact A-scan equipment (contact method)
2) Contact B-scan equipment (contact method)
3) Immersion A- and B-scan equipment
4) Doppler examination equipment

With the contact method, the transducer directly touches the palpebra or sclera and A-scan (A-mode) or B-scan (B-mode) tomography is performed (Figure 1). With the immersion method, the eye is scanned by a transducer in a rubber tank or water tank, with a surgical drape attached in front of the eye (Figure 2). The procedures used for the immersion method can be somewhat complicated. Children, for example, must sometimes be put under general anesthesia. The method does, however, produce better images (Figure 3). With

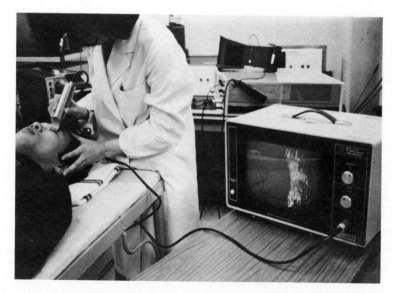

Figure 1. The contact B-scan method by Bronson-Turner Ophthalmic B-scan. The display is a television picture tube.

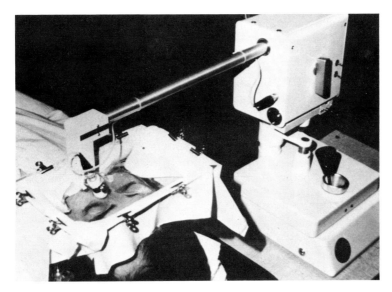

Figure 2. The immersion A- and B-scan method with St. Marianna's high-powered ophthalmic ultrasonic equipment. Mechanical combined scanning is performed while the patient is supine on an examination table. This reduces the patient's head movement and permits the examiner to observe the relationship of transducer to eye while also observing the scan display on the oscilloscope. The scanner arm may be swung into various positions to obtain vertical or oblique scans.

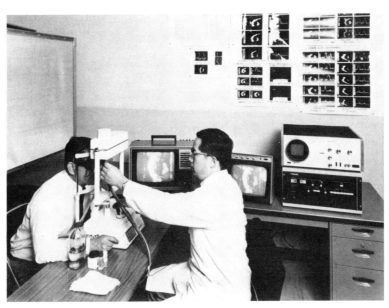

Figure 3. A simplified immersion stand-off system devised by author that allows automatically spaced horizontal scanning.

61

Doppler diagnostic equipment, the rate of blood flow in the intraocular vessels is measured.

DIAGNOSIS OF INTRAOCULAR TUMORS

Retinoblastoma

Retinoblastoma is the most common malignant ocular tumor in children. 100–150 cases are reported annually in Japan. Successful therapy lies in early diagnosis. There is no problem if the tumor can be seen ophthalmoscopically, since it can be diagnosed directly. However, ultrasonic diagnosis is necessary when the tumor is behind a detached retina or when inflammatory vitreous opacities or vitreous hemorrhage are present.

According to Howard (1) and Stafford et al (2), if only standard examination methods are used, this tumor will be falsely diagnosed in 7–14.9% of cases. Oksala et al (3) reported that the A mode characteristics of retinoblastoma resemble organized vitreous hemorrhage. Till et al (4) reported that only 25% of retinoblastomas could be diagnosed correctly.

As has been reported by Sterns et al (5), two morphological types are found in the B scan tomographic images of retinoblastoma, i.e., the solid pattern and the cystic pattern types (Figure 4). In solid B-scan tomographic images, the margin is clear, the internal echo is solid, and the retinoblastoma is continuous with the retina in all sections. In the cystic type, the margin is not always clear, the image contains acoustic vacuoles, and the retinoblastoma is not always continuous with the retina.

The three characteristics common to the solid and cystic patterns are (a) the acoustic attentuation is relatively small (except for tumors with severe calcification), (b) they often lack choroidal excavation and (c) they are accompanied by retinal detachment.

Malignant Choroidal Melanoma

Accurate diagnosis of malignant melanoma is yet to be mastered by the ophthalmologist. The incidence of malignant melanoma is lower in Japan than that in Europe or in the United States. Only about 30 cases are reported annually. Many of these malignant melanomas, however, are in the ocular fundus, and in some cases an accurate diagnosis of an ophthalmoscopically visual focus cannot be made even when ophthalmoscopic examination, scleral indentation, scleral tesselation, fluorescein angiography, visual field examination and radioisotope scintigraphy are used in combination. In such cases, ultrasonic diagnosis is valuable in differentiating solid choroidal tumors from subretinal foci that are filled with serous fluid or blood.

The four choroidal tumors that must be differentiated (since the methods of treating them are different) are malignant choroidal melanoma, metastatic cancer, angioma and subretinal organized hemorrhage (including disciform macular degeneration).

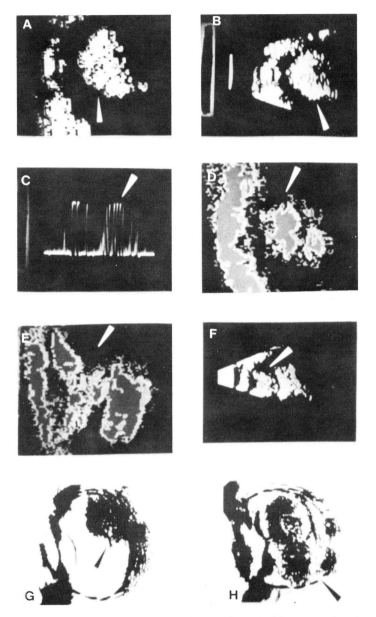

Figure 4. B-scan ultrasonograms of globes with retinoblastoma showing solid and cystic masses. In general, a retinoblastoma has a low-amplitude profile and often resembles the A-scan pattern of vitreous hemorrhage. (*A* and *B*) Solid-type echo pattern of retinoblastoma by digital color display. (*C–F*) Disseminated retinoblastoma in the ocular bulb showing a cystic pattern. (*G*) Solid-echo type pattern. (*H*) Cystic-echo type pattern. (From Tane S and Kimura Y: *Jpn J Ophthalmol* 22:405–411, 1978.)

Malignant melanoma and metastatic cancer are of various sizes; they may be only a protrusion or may occupy almost the entire bulb. Fortunately, they can all be visualized on the B-mode image. In our experience, angiomas rarely protrude more than 5–6 mm but are rather broad horizontally. Subretinal hemorrhage and disciform macular degeneration examined by ultrasonography protrude very little, usually less than 4 mm.

Malignant melanoma shows two characteristic forms, polypoid and convex. Both shapes are clearly and directly visualized by B-scanning. The most common form of malignant melanoma is the elevated solid tumor (Figure 5). In this type, the growth of the lesion is inhibited by the Bruch membrane. In the polypoid (collar-button) type, the tumor breaks the Bruch membrane and appears in the vitreous body. When the scan plane passes through the stem of the tumor, it has a mushroom-like appearance. When the plane does not pass through the stem, it is seen as an isolated disciform mass in the vitreous body (Figure 6). In such cases, serial B-mode tomographic examinations are necessary to trace the site of attachment of the tumor developing from the choroid.

The location of the tumor also helps in distinguishing its type. Angiomas often are found in the posterior region, particularly near the optic nerve disc. Metastatic tumors also are frequently found in the posterior region, but malignant melanomas are found throughout the choroid.

In the B-mode examination, metastatic cancers generally show more rapid growth than malignant melanomas. In metastatic cancer and angioma, the attenuation of the complicated A-mode amplitude echo is lower and flat decay slopes are produced, but the initial amplitude is high. On the other hand, in subretinal hemorrhage and cystic lesions, attenuation is sharp and the acoustic attenuation is high. Malignant melanoma shows an intermediate attenuation curve.

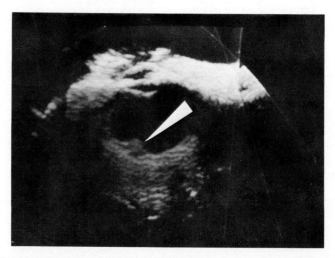

Figure 5. B-scan ultrasonogram of a small malignant melanoma at the posterior pole of the globe, showing an elevation of approximately 3 mm. The presence of choroidal excavation aids in the evaluation of small tumors, but an A-scan through the tumor is required for more precise tissue differentiation. (From Tane S and Kimura Y: *Jpn J Ophthalmol* 22:405–411, 1978.)

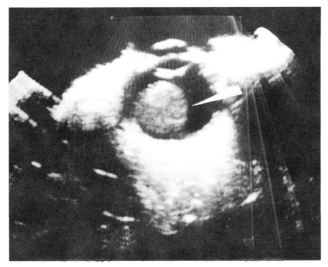

Figure 6. B-scan ultrasonogram of a large intraocular malignant melanoma demonstrating a quiet zone in the posterior aspect of the tumor caused by absorption of sound and tumor homogeneity. (From Tane S and Kimura Y: *Jpn J Ophthalmol* 22:405–411, 1978.)

Ultrasonic characteristics of retinal tumors generally seen in the B-scan ultrasonic images are acoustic vacuoles or quiet zones, choroidal excavation and acoustic shadowing or absorption defects (Figure 7). These are associated with the degree of homogeneity in the tumor, the amount of infiltration by the mass and the extent of acoustic attenuation. With increased frequency, their incidence rises because attenuation increases.

Conditions Simulating Choroidal Tumors

Retinal Lesions.   In retinal detachment or retinoschisis, the ultrasonic pattern may show an elevated vitreoretinal interface echo, but since the subretinal space is sonolucent, the elevation is readily distinguishable from a tumor. Disciform macular degeneration also shows an elevated vitreoretinal interface. These hemorrhagic lesions show low-amplitude internal echoes on A-scan, but will appear hollow at 15 and 20 MHz (or with reduced gain at 10 MHz).

In chorioretinitis, an area of elevated retina may be seen, but the subretinal space is acoustically clear. Retinal pigment epithelium (RPE) lesions (such as congenital hypertrophy of the pigment epithelium) that appear flat and highly pigmented ophthalmoscopically do not have sufficient elevation to be detected ultrasonically.

Choroidal Lesions.   Most benign choroidal nevi are not significantly elevated and therefore cannot be demonstrated on B-scan ultrasonograms. Choroidal detachments present a typical B-scan convex circumferential elevation straddling the ora serrata with a sonolucent area between the retina and sclera. Organized choroidal hemorrhage may be difficult to distinguish acoustically from a tumor, but the internal echoes are of lower amplitude. Lymphoid hyperplasia of the choroid may be ultrasonically indistinguishable from an "en

ACOUSTIC CHARACTERISTICS OF
CHOROIDAL TUMORS

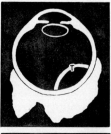

ACOUSTIC
"QUIET ZONE"
(OR "VACUOLE")

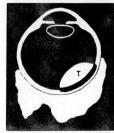

"CHOROIDAL
EXCAVATION"

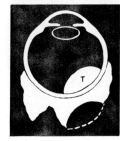

ACOUSTIC
"SHADOWING"
(OR "ABSORPTION DEFECT")

Figure 7. Three types of B-scan texture changes that are useful in the identification of ocular tumors. These morphologic changes are best seen on the two-dimensional B-scan, because they require comparison with adjacent tissues. (Reprinted with permission from Coleman DJ, Lizzi FL, Jack RL: Ultrasonography of the Eye and Orbit. Lea & Febiger, Philadelphia, 1977.)

plaque" melanoma but may be suspected due to greater sound absorption by inflammatory tissue.

Vitreous Lesions.   Vitreous hemorrhages that have undergone organization may appear as acoustically dense masses (Figure 8). In contrast to collar-button melanomas, however, no connecting stalk can be found on serial sectioning, and the internal echo amplitudes are usually lower than those seen in melanoma. The presence of a vitreoretinal interface appearing smoothly curved and in normal position may help in differentiating these hemorrhages. Repeated ultrasonic evaluations may be necessary to distinguish a tumor that lies within a dense vitreous hemorrhage, a situation that arises more often with retinoblastoma than with choroidal tumors. The extremely difficult diagnostic problem of organized hemorrhage in conjunction with retinal detachment arises rarely. The use of varying transducer frequencies, M-mode and quantitative scanning methods may be required to establish the correct diagnosis.

Reliability and Limitations of Ultrasonic Differentiation

The reliability of ultrasonic diagnosis in our laboratory is greater than 96% for differentiation of neoplastic choroidal tumors from benign subretinal hemorrhages, vitreous hemorrhages and retinal detachments. Ossoinig (6) has reported a similar figure.

We have examined nearly 1,000 patients with ocular tumors, both neoplastic and benign. It has not always been possible to identify the tissue present on one examination. Serial examinations are often required to permit growth documentation as well as to repeat the evaluation. The methods described here, even when absolute differentiation cannot be made, can direct the course of treatment. Also, small solid tumors can be followed, patients with larger tumors can benefit from a search for metastatic lesions and ^{32}P scintigraphy tests can be directed to the appropriate area.

In addition to the problems in identifying discrete lesions discussed above, other difficulties in ultrasonic diagnosis of choroidal tumors exist that are related to size or position.

First, very small lesions cannot be demonstrated ultrasonically. In general, lesions causing more than 1 mm of elevation of the retina can be demonstrated, and when the tumor can be visualized and the ultrasonogram is performed under optimal conditions, tumors causing only 0.5 mm of elevation can be depicted. Smaller lesions can certainly be missed with ultrasonography. This is a problem of equivocal significance since there is a growing body of opinion that eyes with small lesions should not be enucleated immediately but rather be followed or treated. It is customary clinically to follow a very small lesion to document a visual growth change. By the time such changes can be documented, the tumor should be demonstrable ultrasonically.

Second, very large lesions filling the vitreous are often confusing in that they may resemble vitreous hemorrhage. In our experience, these tumors have not exhibited choroidal excavation and their A-scan pattern can resemble hemorrhage. This is a particular problem with massive necrotic melanomas and it also occurs with retinoblastoma.

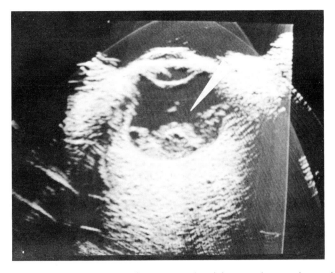

Figure 8. B-scan ultrasonogram of an organized hemorrhage along the posterior limiting membrane of the vitreous. The retina is close to the membrane but is in place. (From Tane S and Kimura Y: *Jpn J Ophthalmol* 22:405–411, 1978.)

Finally, difficulties persist with optimal B-scan visualization of the ora serrata and pars plana regions. Even with the immersion technique, structures that lie perpendicular to the examining beam are well portrayed, but structures lying parallel to the beam, such as the ocular walls at the ora, are not well outlined. Also, structures preceding a tumor will tend to mask some of its acoustic profile. Malignant melanomas seen in this area do not demonstrate choroidal excavation, which makes differentiation more difficult.

Ciliary Body Abnormalities

Ciliary body tumors occur less frequently than tumors of the choroid, accounting for approximately 10% of all ocular melanomas. Tumors of the ciliary body are often difficult to diagnose clinically for they arise in an area of the eye not routinely examined and usually are not amenable to fluorescein angiography. They precipitate cataracts or secondary retinal detachments, which cause difficulty in clinical diagnosis. In addition, ophthalmoscopically visible masses may be difficult to distinguish from cystic lesions of the ciliary body, with elevation of the pigmented epithelium of the ciliary body in this area. Thus, ultrasonography is of great value in the diagnosis of such tumors.

Attention to certain technical features will improve ultrasonic portrayal of ciliary body tumors. First, it is important to rotate the eye as much as possible, bringing the mass perpendicular (in either an anterior or posterior position) to the transducer for best resolution. Second, small tumors in this region may be missed, particularly at the 6:00 and 12:00 meridians, with horizontal scans, so vertical scans are required. Third, a range of transducer frequencies should be used to optimize differentiation. Fourth serial examinations at a later date are necessary in equivocal cases.

Ciliary Body Tumors

The ultrasonographic characteristics of ciliary body tumors will be discussed, as were choroidal tumors, in terms of morphologic and acoustic characteristics.

The location and size of ciliary body tumors can be well demonstrated by B-scan ultrasound. Secondary changes, such as retinal detachment, hemorrhage in the vitreous and cataractous lens changes, can also be shown, as previously discussed.

As in tumors of the choroid, acoustic quiet zones at the posterior part of a ciliary body tumor can be appreciated. We have not had experience with enough ciliary body melanomas to establish the significance of frequency-related variation; however, the quiet zone phenomenon is best seen at high transducer frequencies. Choroidal excavation has not been seen with ciliary body tumors, and thus this useful differential sign is not available.

Lesions Simulating Ciliary Body Tumors

B scan ultrasonography provides differential diagnosis between ciliary body cysts and ciliary body tumors. The interior of the cyst is sonolucent, and the A-scan trace remains at baseline throughout the cyst. A B-scan ultrasonogram of a patient with a ciliary body cyst demonstrates the obviously cystic structure of the lesion.

Choroidal detachments or effusions can simulate a ring melanoma of the ciliary body, but ultrasonography can demonstrate their cystic or solid natures.

Usefulness of Ultrasound in Diagnosing Ciliary Body Tumors

Ciliary body tumors are often misdiagnosed. In one series, 40% of misdiagnoses were due to obscuration by retinal or choroidal detachment, and 5% were misinterpreted as cystic lesions. Ultrasonography can improve the differential diagnosis, even in patients with clear media. The size and the posterior extent of these tumors, as determined by serial acoustic tomography, influence a decision regarding corneoscleral iridocyclectomy. The clinician can often fail to appreciate the position of the posterior edge of the tumor with ophthalmoscopic or slit-lamp examination techniques, even in the presence of clear media, whereas ultrasonography can show this variable.

We do not have enough experience to differentiate melanomas from metastatic tumors in this area by quantitative A-scan ultrasonography. Metastatic tumors, however, are quite unusual in a position anterior to the ora serrata. Ordinarily, a metastatic tumor can be diagnosed clinically on the basis of multiple tumors, known primary tumor, and relatively rapid growth.

DIAGNOSIS OF ORBITAL TUMORS

Purnell (7) and Coleman (8) divided orbital tumor images by B-scan tomography into the following categories on the basis of their sound transmission: cystic tumors with good sound transmission and clear rounded margins, angiomatous tumors with good sound transmission and irregular margins, solid tumors with poor transmission and rounded margins, and infiltrative tumors with poor transmission and irregular margins. This classification is a practical and valuable method for clinical diagnosis (Figure 9).

Cystic Lesions

Paranasal Mucocele

Paranasal mucoceles often appear on the upper or inner wall of the orbit and cause the orbit to deviate downward or outward (Figure 10). Bone defects aid in the diagnosis of mucoceles by simple x-ray examination, but they are sometimes difficult to detect. CT scanning is valuable in the morphological identification of mucoceles.

B-scan tomography of a cystic tumor shows a cystic image with a clear, smooth margin, an elevated outline and the orbital fat pressed aside. The pus and mucus in the tumor transmits sound well, and the anterior wall of the mucocele can be well visualized. The contents produce no echo, but there are several weak echos of low amplitude due to the waste products of the contents.

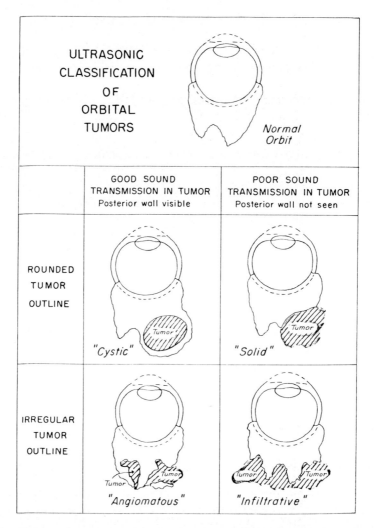

Figure 9.   Schematic presentation of the division of orbital tumor patterns based on their outline and transmission properties. (Reprinted with permission from Coleman DJ, Lizzi FL, Jack RL: Ultrasonography of the Eye and Orbit. Lea & Febiger, Philadelphia, 1977.)

Solid Lesions

Lesions showing this echo pattern are mainly primary neurogenic tumors. Glioma arise from the optic nerve, neurofibroma and neurilemmona arise from around the optic nerves and meningioma (echo pattern to be discussed below) infiltrates from an intracranial lesion (Figure 11).

The characteristics of the B-mode tomographic images of these lesions are as follows: Inside the muscle cone these tumors show a solid tumor echo pattern, the W-shaped orbital fat tissue is deformed by pressure from the tumor, and the orbit may be excavated. The lesion is disciform and solid with a clear

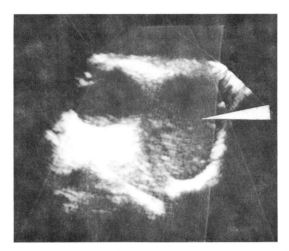

Figure 10. B-scan ultrasonogram of a large orbital mucocele showing a rounded anterior border and good outlining of the orbital wall. Slight compression of the globe anterior to the tumor can be seen. (From Tane S and Kimura Y: *Jpn J Ophthalmol* 22:405–411, 1978.)

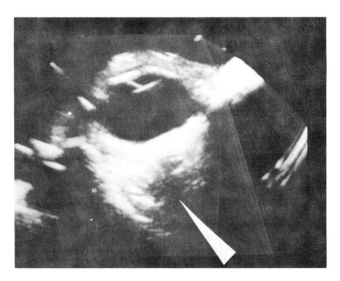

Figure 11. B-scan ultrasonogram of a glioma of the optic nerve. Both glioma and meningioma appear as a solid tumor in the region of the optic nerve, producing a marked widening of the normal nerve shadow. This tumor appears sonolucent, indicating marked homogeneity. The enlargement of the nerve sheath and displacement of the adjacent orbital fat indicate a neurogenic tumor. (From Tane S and Kimura Y: *Jpn J Ophthalmol* 22:405–411, 1978.)

margin, and absorbed-sound attenuation is moderate; thus, the posterior margin shows acoustic vacuoles and is often not clearly visible. The inside reflection scatters an interrupted medium amplitude echo due to the alveolar construction of the cells inside the tumor and to the presence of the middle septum and blood vessels, that is, it shows a heterogeneous solid B-scan echo pattern. Sometimes a negative echo for the optic nerve is replaced by this pattern.

Angiomatous Lesions

Hemangiomas

Hemangiomas occur in all parts of the orbit, including the inner and outer part of the muscle cone or optic accessory organs. The most frequently occurring intraorbital angiomatous tumors, cavernous hemangioma, consist of small vacuoles filled with blood and a fibrous septum. Sound transmission is good. Therefore, the inside echo is produced by the entire tumor and has a heterogeneous high amplitude not accompanied by attenuation; this is in contrast to the attenuated medium-amplitude echo seen in solid tumors. The B mode tomographic image has a clear margin because the lesion is surrounded by a peculiar capsule (Figure 12). An echo image of secondary changes due to pressure from the tumor, such as depression of orbit and orbital fat, dislocation of the optic nerve and choked disc, are sometimes observed.

Infiltrative Lesions

Lymphomas

Lymphomas range from benign to malignant, most gradually increase in size, and the site of their occurrence in the orbit varies. They are found even in such locations as the muscle cone, the lacrimal gland and along the orbital bony wall. B-mode tomography shows a solid, infiltrative image for most. Since the lesion is solid, sound transmission is poor, inner echos with medium amplitude are produced, and the anterior rim of the tumor is often not clear (acoustic vacuole) due to absorbed-sound attenuation. The outline of the lymphoma is irregular because it has no capsule, and B-mode tomography shows an infiltrative image. Some benign lymphomas, which have a solid inner structure, lack a middle septum, are heterogeneous, have clear margins and may be mistaken for cystic lesions, but they can be differentiated since lymphomas greatly attenuate sound (Figure 13).

Sarcomas and Metastatic Tumors

Both primary and secondary sarcomas produce ultrasonic images similar to those of other infiltrative tumors (poor sound transmission, irregular margin). Secondary tumors infiltrating the orbit from the paranasal cavity tend to spread along the orbital wall outside the muscle cone, whereas rhabdomyosarcomas originating in the orbit are first localized on the inside or outside

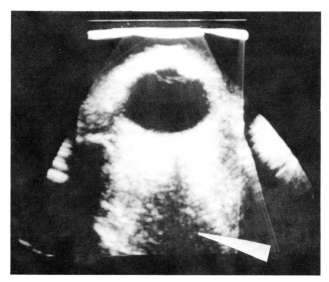

Figure 12. B-scan ultrasonogram of an orbital hemangioma. The relatively rounded anterior surface, good sound transmission properties and overall size of the mass are demonstrated. (From Tane S and Kimura Y: *Jpn J Ophthalmol* 22:405–411, 1978.)

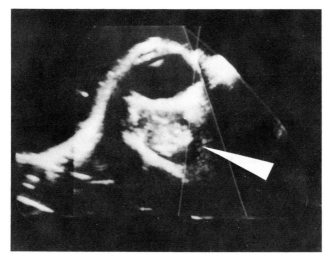

Figure 13. B-scan ultrasonogram of a malignant lymphoma extending into the orbital fat, demonstrating a relatively poor transmission pattern and extensions of the tumor into adjacent areas. (From Tane S and Kimura Y: *Jpn J Ophthalmol* 22:405–411, 1978.)

of the muscle cone, later spreading into other spaces and showing an echo pattern characteristic of infiltrative tumors (Figure 14).

Meningiomas

Meningiomas spread from the skull cavity to the inside of the orbit. When a meningioma includes the optic nerve, it shows an echo pattern similar to that of optic nerve tumors, and when it infiltrates along the orbital wall it does not show focal morphology and becomes difficult to visualize ultrasonographically. When secondary congestive changes occur in the orbit, these lesions may be falsely diagnosed as congestive or inflammatory lesions, as will be discussed later. Diagnosis should be made by combining ultrasonographic examination with x-ray examination and, in particular, CT scan.

Pseudotumors

The mass lesion type of orbital pseudotumor presents an ultrasonographic appearance which is similar to the infiltrative tumor pattern discussed. This is a difficult area for ultrasonic differential diagnosis. The typical patterns seen acoustically in orbital pseudotumors is an irregular notching of the orbital fat by a sonolucent mass. Inflammatory granulomas absorb sound to such a degree that internal echos are not usually seen.

Lacrimal Gland Tumors

Tumors of the lacrimal gland can be benign or highly neoplastic. Benign pseudotumors are confined to the gland, although inflammation may invade adjoining muscle. Adenocarcinoma or squamous carcinoma involving the lacrimal gland may invade other tissues. Since only the anterior tip of these tumors

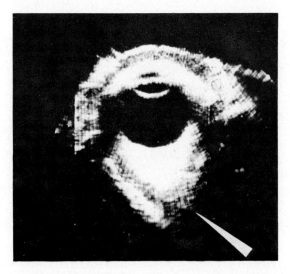

Figure 14.   B-scan ultrasonogram of a metastatic carcinoma with irregular outline and relatively poor sound transmission. (From Tane S and Kimura Y: *Jpn J Ophthalmol* 22:405–411, 1978.)

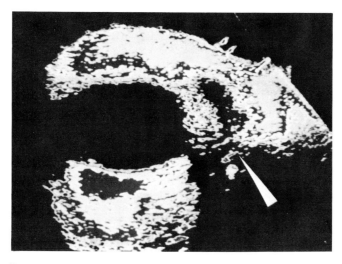

Figure 15. B-scan color-coding ultrasonogram of lacrimal gland tumor showing indentation of the normal palpebra and orbital fat pattern. Localized tumors of this type are usually best evaluated by a contact A-scan technique, since the ultrasonic beam can be more precisely directed. Extensions of a lacrimal gland tumor are better seen on the B-scan display, because it allows accentuation of the orbital wall and indentation of the orbital fat to be portrayed. (From Tane S and Kimura Y: *Jpn J Ophthalmol* 22:405–411, 1978.)

can be palpated, ultrasonography is useful in determining the size, extent and configuration of tumors in this area.

Lacrimal gland tumors generally appear as solid tumors with well-demonstrated contours, poor sound transmission and few internal echoes. Their size and shape are highly variable, and, because of bony overhang from the superior orbital rim, they may not be easily outlined with B scan. Ultrasonic evaluation is most useful in determining the posterior extension of the tumor and the lateral enlargement of invading orbital tissue (Figure 15). This finding indicates a malignant lesion.

It is best to use contact A scan techniques to complete the evaluation of the lacrimal gland area.

SUMMARY

Ultrasonography is a valuable tool in the morphological diagnosis of lesions in the eye and surrounding tissues. A- and B-scanning methods, with immersion, have better resolution and better diagnostic precision than contact methods, whereas automatic mechanical scanning minimizes differences in the skill of the user and produces reproducible results. On the other hand, the contact scanners are less complicated and more easily applied and, ideally, both types of instrument should be employed in major diagnostic centers.

REFERENCES

1. Howard GM: Erroneous clinical diagnosis of retinoblastoma and uveal melanoma. Trans Am Acad Ophthalmol Otolaryngol 73: 199, 1969.
2. Stafford WR, Yanoff M, Parnell BL: Retinoblastoma initially misdiagnosed as primary ocular inflammation. Arch Ophthalm 82: 771, 1969.
3. Oksala A: The echogram in retinoblastoma. Acta Ophthalmol 37: 132–137, 1959.
4. Till P, Ossoinig K: Echography of retinoblastoma. Ber Dtsch Ophthalmol Ges 69: 203–209, 1969.
5. Sterns GK, Coleman DJ, Ellsworth RM: The ultrasonographic characteristics of retinoblastoma. Am J Ophthalmol 78: 606–611, 1974.
6. Ossoinig K, Till P: Methods and results of ultrasonography in diagnosing intraocular tumors. In Gitser K, et al (ed): Ophthalmic Ultrasound. St. Louis, CV Mosby Co, 1969, pp 294–300.
7. Purnell, E.W.: Ultrasound in ophthalmological diagnosis. In Grossman C, et al (ed): Ophthalmic Ultrasound. New York, Plenum Press. 1969, pp 95–109.
8. Coleman DJ, Lizzi FL, Jack RL: Ultrasonography of the Eye and Orbit. Philadelphia, Lea & Febiger, 1977, pp 213–244.
9. Tane S, Kimura Y: Ultrasonic characteristics of retinoblastoma. Jap J Ophthalmol 22: 405–411, 1978.
10. Tane S, Kimura Y: The development and clinical application of the high-powered ophthalmic B-scan equipment. In Gernet H (ed): Diagnostica ultrasonica in Ophthalmologica: Proceedings of SIDUO-VII, Meeting, R.M. Remy Verlag, Munster, 1978, pp 8–11.
11. Tane S: Tomographic reconstruction of the reflectivity image. In Wagai T, Omoto R (eds): Ultrasound in Medicine and Biology (Proceedings of 2-WFUMB), Amsterdam, Excerpta Medica, 1980, pp 94–100.
12. Tane S, Yamamoto Y: Echographic Diagnosis and Its Therapy in Ophthalmology. (In Japanese). Tokyo, Kanehara Shuppan, 1972.

6

ECHOGRAPHIC DIAGNOSIS OF TUMORS OF THE THYROID GLAND

Toshio Wagai

The first results of echographic imaging of the thyroid gland were reported by Howry (1). He developed the special water-bag mechanical compound scanner, "Somascope," and succeeded in obtaining clear images of the thyroid gland in a complete cross-sectional echogram of the neck. Soon after, Wagai (2, 3) and other Japanese investigators (4) reported their results. Interesting results were also described by Damascelli et al (5), Thijis (6), Rasmussen et al (7), Blum et al (8), and Miskin et al (9). All these investigators used a simple mechanical immersion scanner and manual-contact scanning technique, which were developed for the echographic imaging of the breast and the abdomen. This type of equipment is not well suited for the examination of small, anatomically complex organs such as the thyroid, and this unfavorably affected the quality of the images. Weill (10) utilized a mechanical real-time scanner for the investigation of the thyroid gland and proved the effectiveness of real-time scanning in this field. Jellins et al (11) applied the specially developed gray scale echographic technique in this field and recorded clear cross-sectional echographic images of thyroid lesions. I have attempted to develop equipment that may be utilized for imaging both the breast and the thyroid gland and in this paper will describe the echographic images of the normal thyroid and pathological conditions of the thyroid gland obtained with this equipment. Criteria for differentiating thyroid gland disease, particularly benign and malignant nodular goiter, will also be discussed (12, 13).

INSTRUMENTATION FOR ECHOGRAPHIC IMAGING OF THE THYROID GLAND

In 1965, I first attempted to image the thyroid gland with equipment used for the detection of breast tumors. This instrument employed simple linear scanning and a water-bag system. Unfortunately, the results were not encouraging because of the poor performance of the equipment. Then I applied simple linear

77

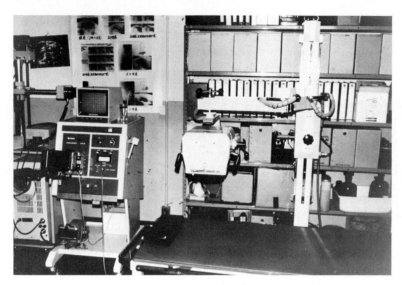

Figure 1. Echographic equipment for scanning the breast.

and mechanical compound scanning techniques and finally, with the development of the gray scale display technique in 1968, obtained good echographic images of the thyroid gland. The equipment developed at our research center mainly for imaging breast tissue is illustrated in Figure 1; the method for performing a transverse scan of the thyroid is shown in Figure 2. Simple mechanical linear scanning is used, and coupling of the energy is achieved with a watertight bag. The length of the scan is 15 cm and the depth of the water in the water bag is 5–10 cm. This is sufficient to image the whole thyroid gland. A 5-MHz focused PZT transducer 10 mm in diameter and 80 mm in

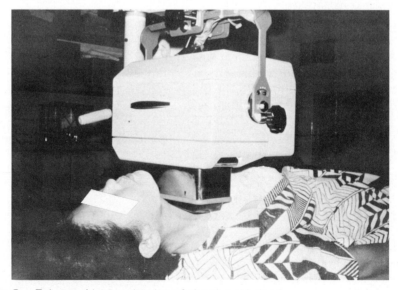

Figure 2. Echographic examination of the thyroid gland.

radius is used. Recently, a polyvinylidene fluoride (PVDF) transducer also gave good results. The scanning speed is 2 seconds, the scanning area is 15 × 5 cm, and serial parallel echography at any desired interval may be recorded. A dynamic wide-range amplifier with approximately 80 dB and a short-life cathode-ray tube (CRT) with sharp spots are used for photographing the echograms, and a long-life CRT or television monitor using a scan conversion system is used as a monitor. The system is compact and echographic examination of the thyroid gland and breast are easily performed.

ECHOGRAPHIC IMAGES OF NORMAL THYROID AND BENIGN NODULAR GOITER

Figure 3 is an example of a transverse echogram of the normal thyroid gland obtained with the equipment. With improvements in resolution and development of gray scale, the anatomical structure of the thyroid gland, neck vessels and neck muscles is clearly demonstrated.

Figure 4 is an example of nine serial parallel echograms of a normal thyroid taken at 5-mm intervals. These serial echograms are produced within 30 seconds and show that the whole thyroid gland may be examined in a short time. Echographic images of the normal thyroid gland (Figure 5) differ slightly in size and shape according to the patient's age and other factors. Nevertheless, the normal thyroid is clearly outlined and is seen to contain a uniform distribution of weak fine internal echoes. In hyperthyroidism (Figure 6), the swelling and enlargement of the thyroid gland together with the fine internal ho-

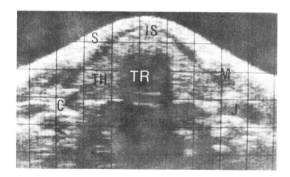

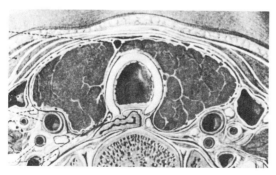

Figure 3. Transverse image of the normal thyroid gland. S:skin; Is: isthmus; TH: thyroid; C: carotid artery; J: jugular vein; TR: trachea; M: muscle layers.

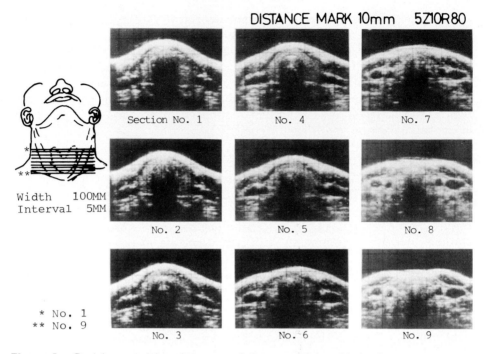

DISTANCE MARK 10mm   5Z10R80

Section No. 1   No. 4   No. 7

No. 2   No. 5   No. 8

No. 3   No. 6   No. 9

Width   100MM
Interval   5MM

* No. 1
** No. 9

Figure 4.   Serial grey scale echograms of the normal thyroid gland.

mogeneous echo content is easily recognized. Measurement of the maximum depth at the isthmus, of both lobes and of the maximum width of the thyroid gland are easily carried out. Figure 7 is an example of nine serial echograms of hyperthyroidism taken at 5-mm intervals. By this procedure, not only can the whole thyroid gland be echographically examined but its volume also can be measured. This technique is superior to the usual Allen-Goodwin method, which uses scintigraphy. Measurement of thyroid gland volume is important, particularly for following and estimating the clinical effect of conservative treatment of hyperthyroidism. Manual-contact scanning has been used by many investigators for imaging the thyroid. The improvement in instrumentation has brought about a reevaluation of contact scanning. Figure 8 is a scan of hyperthyroidism obtained by modern contact scanning equipment operating at 5 MHz and using a digital scan converter. The image is clear but the method still has a problem providing reproducible images and suffers from the complexity of the scanning procedure.

Differentiation of benign and malignant nodular goiters is most important from the clinical point of view. Simple palpation, x-ray examination, scintigraphy and, recently, x-ray computed tomography are used for this purpose. At the same time, echographic imaging, with its ability to visualize soft tissue, is also being employed. The criteria developed at our research center for differentiating benign and malignant nodular goiters are shown in Figure 9. Benign and malignant nodular goiters show cystic degeneration more often than do breast tumors, and this can cause difficulty in differentiation. It has been found useful to divide echographic images of nodular goiter into two

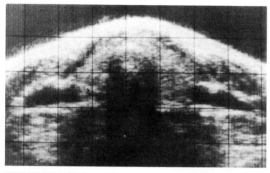

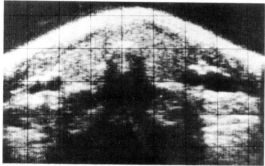

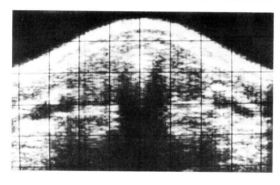

Figure 5.   Echographic images of normal thyroid gland. Mechanical linear scan, 5 MHz.

groups, the solid type and the cyst-forming type. Figure 10 shows four cases of benign nodular goiter (adenoma) of the solid type. Echographic differentiation of benign goiter of the solid type is relatively easy. The margin of the tumor is smooth and the internal area is filled by a weak, fine homogeneous echo pattern. Figure 11 is an example of nine serial echograms of adenoma (the same case shown in Figure 10A) taken at 5-mm intervals. Problems are ecnountered with the cyst-forming type. Benign adenomas, particularly follicular adenoma, often show cystic degeneration. Assessment of cyst-forming adenomas requires high-quality imaging. Figure 12 is a comparison of the scintigram and echogram of a follicular adenoma with cystic degeneration. The scintigram shows only defect of radioisotope (RI) in the upper pole of the left lobe and in the lower part of the right lobe, whereas the echogram shows a clear image of cystic degeneration in the same areas and a diffuse adenoma image in the lower part of the right lobe. Echograph also is helpful as a guide in needle aspiration biopsy. Figure 13 shows four cases of adenoma with cystic

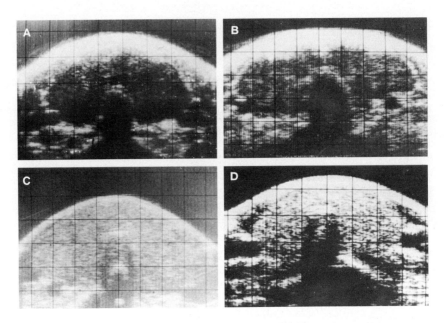

Figure 6. Echographic images of hyperthyroidism, 5 MHz.

DISTANCE MARK 10 mm   5 Z10R80

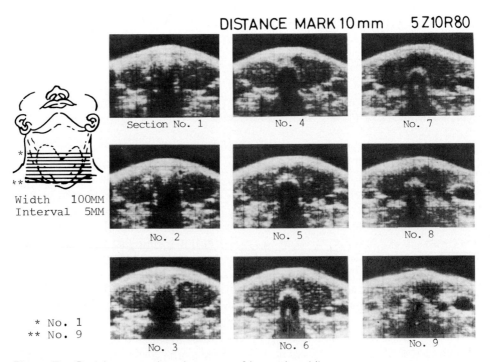

Width   100MM
Interval   5MM

Section No. 1   No. 4   No. 7
No. 2   No. 5   No. 8
No. 3   No. 6   No. 9

* No. 1
** No. 9

Figure 7. Serial grey scale echograms of hyperthyroidism.

82

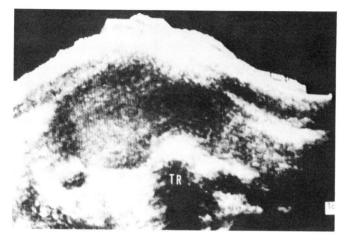

Figure 8.   Echogram of hyperthyroidism obtained by contact scanning, 5 MHz.

degeneration. In the early stage of cystic change (Figure 13A), small multiple cystic images with smooth and punched-out margins are seen. With advance in cystic change, an almost cystic appearance is obtained. The little remaining tissue has a fine, homogeneous echo content (Figure 13B). In more advanced cystic change, a pure cystic image is obtained (Figure 13C and D). Figure 14 shows nine serial echograms of the case seen in Figure 13C taken at 5-mm intervals. Visualization of the remaining tissues facilitates the differentiation

Medical Ultrasonics Research Center, Juntendo University

		benign appearance	malignant appearance
solid type	contour, margin	regular (smooth)	strong, irregular
	internal echo content	weak - uniform	ununiform or weak - uniform
cystic formation type	margin of cystic structure	regular (smooth)	irregular irregular prominence circumscribed cystic formation

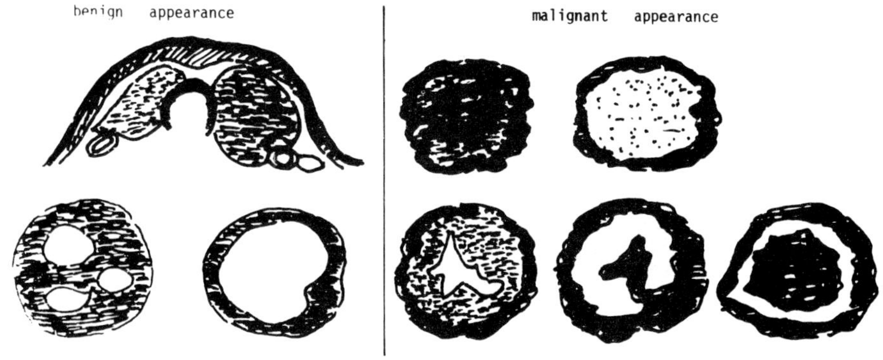

benign appearance   malignant appearance

Figure 9.   Criteria for investigation of echographic thyroid tumor images.

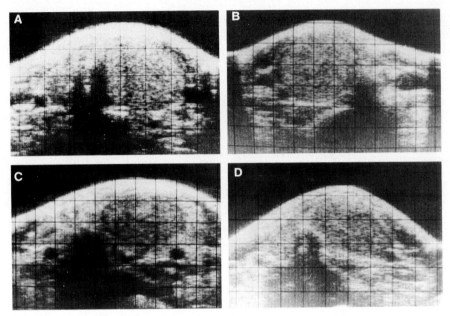

Figure 10. Echograms of a benign nodular goiter (adenoma), 5 MHz.

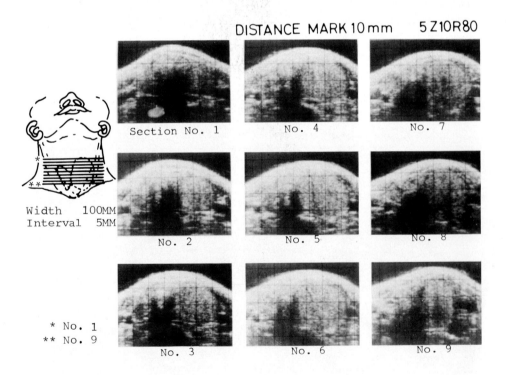

DISTANCE MARK 10 mm   5 Z10R80

Section No. 1   No. 4   No. 7

No. 2   No. 5   No. 8

No. 3   No. 6   No. 9

Width   100MM
Interval   5MM

* No. 1
** No. 9

Figure 11. Grey scale echograms of nodular goiter (adenoma).

84

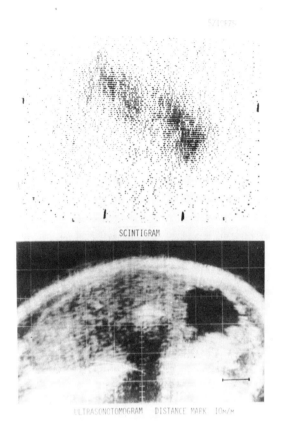

SCINTIGRAM

ULTRASONOTOMOGRAM   DISTANCE MARK 10m/m

Figure 12. Scintigram and ultra-sonotomogram of cystic degeneration of follicular thyroid adenoma.

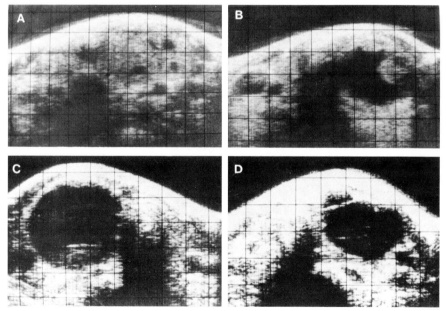

Figure 13. Echographic images of adenoma with cystic degeneration.

85

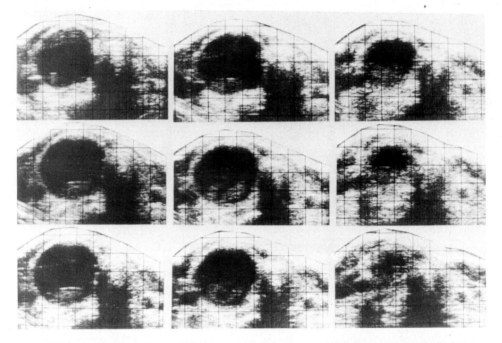

Figure 14. Serial echograms of the case shown in Figure 13c, 3 mm interval, 5 MHz.

of adenoma from a pure cyst. When irregularity is seen in the margins of cystic changes and in the remaining tissue, malignant transformation of benign adenoma must be considered.

ECHOGRAPHIC IMAGES OF THYROID GLAND CARCINOMA

Thyroid gland carcinoma generally presents a more complicated appearance. Thyroid gland carcinoma, which belongs to the solid type, is easily differentiated. Four cases of thyroid gland carcinoma of the solid type are shown in Figure 15. Each reveals irregular margins and irregular tumor internal echo content, which are two of the most characteristic appearances of malignancy. Figure 16 also shows solid-type carcinoma images. In these cases, the irregular internal echo content (Figure 16A) and irregular strong margin of the tumor images have the characteristic malignant appearance. The inside area of the tumor, however, has a fine homogeneous echo pattern (Figure 16B) or an almost cystic appearance (Figure 16C). The relationship between echographic images and the histological structure of thyroid carcinoma is presently under review. The differentiation of malignant appearance requires consideration of all the criteria shown in Figure 7. The problems are the same as with the benign goiter of the cyst-forming type. A characteristic feature of thyroid carcinoma with cystic change is that it is more complex. The most striking characteristic is the irregular shape of the cystic image, as shown in Figure 16C. This case was first thought to be benign adenoma, but with serial echography,

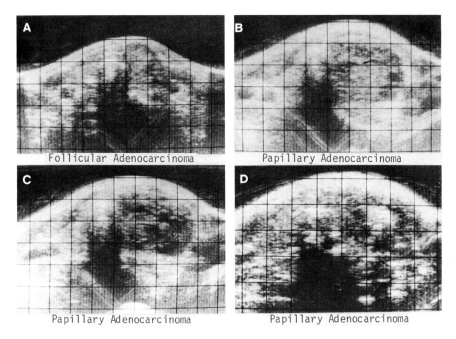

Figure 15. Echograms of thyroid gland carcinoma, 5 MHz.

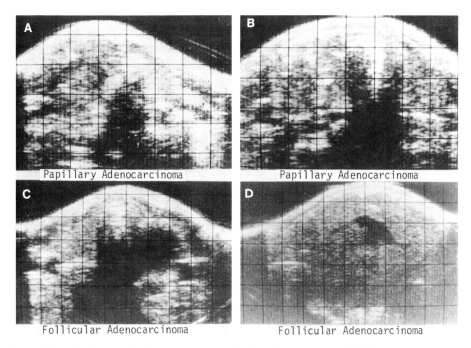

Figure 16. Echographic images of thyroid gland carcinoma, 5 MHz.

87

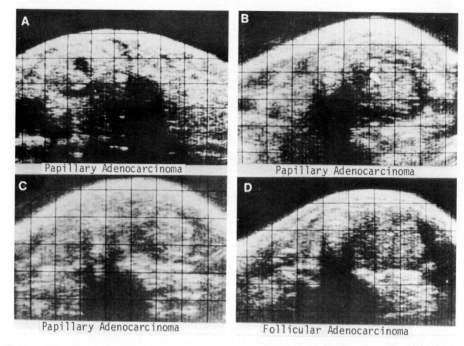

Figure 17. Echographic images of thyroid gland carcinoma with cystic change.

a small cystic image with irregular shape was detected in the middle part of the goiter and malignancy was suspected. Figure 17 shows four cases of thyroid carcinoma with cystic change. The characteristic images of cystic formation in thyroid carcinoma are irregular shape of the cystic images and circumscribed cystic formation in which cystic images are detected mainly in the peripheral part of the tumor (halo sign) and irregularly prominent solid images in the cystic area.

DIAGNOSTIC ACCURACY OF NODULAR GOITER BY ECHOGRAPHY

At our research center, thyroid disease has been examined by biochemical function tests, x-ray, scintigraphy, echography and aspiration biopsy. Table 1

TABLE 1. Ultrasonic Diagnosis of Thyroid Gland Tumors (Juntendo University Hospital, 1973–1980)

Number of Cases (Biopsy)	Physical Examination Scintigraphy X-ray Examination		Echography	
Cancer 72	Malignant	42 (58%)	Malignant	53 (74%)
	Benign	30 (42%)	Benign	19 (26%)
Benign goiter 132	Benign	99 (75%)	Benign	111 (84%)
	Suspected malignant	33 (25%)	Suspected malignant	21 (16%)

gives the results obtained during the last 7 years. The echography results given are those obtained since the new equipment has been used. Accuracy in diagnosing thyroid carcinoma (72 cases) was 74%, which is better than that obtained from other examinations, which showed a 58% diagnostic accuracy. The false-positive rate for benign goiter was 16% in 132 cases, lower than that of other examination techniques, which showed 25%. Integration of all imaging techniques results in the most accurate diagnosis. We can expect improvement of echographic techniques and instrumentation, resulting in more effective echographic imaging, and, thus, in spite of the development of other modes of tissue imaging such as x-ray computed tomography, RCT, nuclear magnetic resonance and digital radiography, echography will continue to be a valuable diagnostic aid.

REFERENCES

1. Howry DH: Techniques used in ultrasonic visualization of soft tissue. In Ultrasound in Biology and Medicine. Washington, DC, American Institute of Biological Science, 1957, p 56.
2. Wagai T, Ishihara A: The application of ultrasonic method for the disease of thyroid with special reference to the measurement of thyroid volume. Jpn Med Ultrason 3: 16, 1965.
3. Wagai T, Tanaka K, Kikuchi Y, et al: Ultrasonic diagnosis in Japan. In Diagnostic Ultrasound, Proceedings of The First International Conference. New York, Plenum Press, 1966, p 27.
4. Fujimoto Y, Oka A, Omoto R, et al: Ultrasound scanning for the thyroid as a new diagnostic approach. Ultrasonics 5: 177, 1967.
5. Damascelli B, Cascinelli N, Livraghi T, et al: Preoperative approach to thyroid tumors by a two-dimensional pulsed echo technique. Ultrasonics 6: 242, 1968.
6. Thijis LG: Diagnostic ultrasound in clinical thyroid investigation. J Clin Endocrinol Metab 32: 709, 1971.
7. Rasmussen SN, Christiansen NJB, Jorgensen JS, et al: Differentiation between cystic and solid thyroid nodules by ultrasonic examination. Acta Chir Scand 137: 331, 1971.
8. Blum M, Goldman AB, Herskovic A, et al: Clinical applications of thyroid echography. N Engl J Med 287: 1164, 1972.
9. Miskin M, Rosen IB, Walfish PG: B-mode ultrasonography in assessment of thyroid gland lesions. Ann Intern Med 79: 505, 1973.
10. Weill F: Clinical Atlas of Ultrasonic Radiography. Paris, Masson & C. Editeurs, 1973.
11. Jellins, J, Kossoff G, Wiseman J, et al: Ultrasonic grey scale visualization of the thyroid gland. Ultrasound Med Biol 1: 405, 1975.
12. Wagai T, Ishihara A, Kobayashi S: Diagnostic ultrasound in thyroid and salivary gland. In Donald I, Levi S (eds): Present and Future of Diagnostic Ultrasound. Rotterdam, Kooyker Scientific Publications, 1977, p 176.
13. Wagai T.: Analysis of echographic thyroid gland carcinoma images. In Kurjak A, Kratochwil A (eds): Recent Advances in Ultrasound Diagnosis 3. Amsterdam, Excerpta Medica, 1981, p 359.

7

ULTRASONIC DIAGNOSIS OF MALIGNANT TUMORS OF THE BREAST

Joan Croll

Work on the sonographic appearance of breast tissue and breast tumors in Australia was begun by Kossoff, Reeve and Jellins in the Ultrasonic Research Section of the Commonwealth Acoustic Laboratories in 1966. At this time, a dedicated waterbath scanner with a 2 MHz transducer was used. Grey scale echography was incorporated in 1969, and in 1974 the frequency of the transducer was changed to 4 MHz. The Ultrasonic Research Section later became the Ultrasonics Institute, and at this Institute, work into the visualization of breast tissue and breast tumors is continuing. The original work performed and the observations made by these Australian workers have become the yardstick for all other workers interested in the ultrasonic characterization of breast tumors.

Instruments designed for general ultrasonography, such as the Ultrasound Institute (Ausonics, Sydney, Australia) (UI) Octoson, are now in use for the ultrasonic visualization of breast tissue, and several small-parts scanners are available with varying qualities of grey scale resolution.

The problem in the interpretation of the breast echogram lies in the inherent differences among breasts. The relative components of fat, active glandular tissue, fibrous tissue and ducts are different in each patient, and vary with the stages in each patient's life and reproductive history. For example, the teenage nulliparous breast is uniformly composed of ducts lying within a fibrous stroma, with very little subcutaneous fat. After a first live birth at an early age, however, the young breast shows fatty infiltration, which increases with each subsequent birth, leaving less active glandular element. The elderly nulliparous breast usually is composed of marked periductal fibrosis, which is readily recognized ultrasonically, and the breast of the elderly primipara, having a first child at age 28 or older, shows similar changes. Gross dysplasia or fibrocystic "disease," which is a process common in women aged 35–55 years, presents a different picture again, and each variation in these "normal" patients has a recognizable series of ultrasonic changes.

The internal echo content of benign and malignant tumors is confusingly

90

alike, and additional information is required if a correct sonographic diagnosis is to be made. Furthermore, the echo pattern of fatty tissue is very similar in amplitude to the echo pattern of both benign and malignant tumors. Thus, apart from an obvious mass, the sonographic determination of malignancy depends on subtle skin changes, disturbances of architecture and surrounding structures within the breast and changes in posterior detail on simple scanning. The presence of a mass containing low-level echoes with an irregular outline is suspicious, but when a skin dimple or protrusion or disruption of pectoral fascia also is found, the diagnosis of carcinoma may be made with greater confidence.

FALSE-NEGATIVE ULTRASONOGRAPHY (TABLE 1)

Ultrasonography is most accurate in mammographically dense breast tissue. It therefore is an ideal complement to mammography because mammography is least accurate in dense breast tissue. Conversely, ultrasonography frequently fails to demonstrate a mass lesion in a fatty breast, despite an obvious clinical and mammographic cancer, because the echoes recorded from such tumors are similar in amplitude to those recorded from fatty tissue.

In an investigative breast clinic the complementary roles of these two tests is established by following up the patients examined and comparing the accuracy of each test reported after the results of biopsy or other further investigations are known. False negative and false positive reports are equally important. To miss a cancer is the most undesirable, but to call more than two or three lesions suspicious when biopsy proves them to be benign for each one cancer correctly reported is at best an expensive way to practice medicine.

TABLE 1. False-negative Sonograms and Mammograms Compared with the Mammographic Appearance of Parenchyma in 186 Patients with Proven Breast Cancer

Parenchyma	24 False-negative Mammograms, 13%*	32 False-negative Sonograms, 17%
Atrophic	8%	56%
Mild dysplasia	42%	23%
Marked dysplasia	25%	9%
Moderate ductal	17%	3%
Marked ductal	8%	9%
	100%	100%

* The false-negative mammography rate in the SSDBC is 9%. All patients with false-negative mammograms are routinely examined by sonography, but not all patients with positive mammograms are examined by sonography. Hence, there is a bias in the figures given above.

Experience in mammography makes the interpretation of breast echography easier, and, at the Sydney Square Diagnostic Breast Clinic (SSDBC), ultrasonography is not performed without adequate and recent mammography, except in women under 25 years of age or during pregnancy and lactation. In this multidisciplinary investigative clinic, women under 25 years of age are examined by a surgeon and by ultrasonography with the UI Octoson. Women over 25 are examined by a surgeon and by routine film-screen mammography. Ultrasonography is added if the breasts are mammographically dense, and/or if there is a clinical or mammographic mass or area of suspicion. Fine-needle aspiration of cysts or fine-needle aspiration biopsy of solid lesions for cytological examination is performed when indicated.

Echography is performed with a UI Octoson used only for breast work which is equipped with 4-MHz transducers. The patient is greeted by the sonographer who palpates both breasts and takes a history of breast problems. Any scars from previous surgery and/or skin lesions are noted diagramatically. After explaining the details of the examination, neutral detergent solution is sponged onto the skin to reduce surface tension and the patient is positioned so that the entire breast is immersed in the waterbath, which is kept at a constant temperature of 35°C. Usually, the left breast is examined first so that the patient is able to observe the screen, which helps allay her anxiety. Patient relaxation is essential inasmuch as movement disturbs the clarity of images. The instrument settings, such as gain and transmit gain control, are set on a transverse scan through the nipple. A scale factor is indicated on the echograms, which are generally taken on a 1.5:1 ratio. The transducer arm is moved then to the upper limit of breast tissue. Using compound scans, sections through the breast are taken at 5-mm intervals to the lower limit of breast tissue. Areas of interest are noted, and sections as small as 1-mm are taken through these areas. Simple scans are performed after the area has been redefined. Images are recorded on 9-format film with a Dunn (model 149) camera. Rotation markers are placed through areas of interest, and the gantry is turned 90° to take sections at right angles. Simple scans from various angles are conducted through the areas of interest; a tilt ability is used to direct the sound wave behind the nipple area. The examination takes a minimum of 20 minutes, and longer if particular attention is paid to a certain area. In the SSDBC, to save time, routine sagittal cuts of the unaffected breast are not performed. We rely on our sonographer to be alert to an area of suspicion during the routine transverse scans. It is generally thought that this is not the best procedure, but our experience has shown it to be practical for our purposes.

Compression of the breast during examination has recently been introduced for patients with a dense, poorly written central breast cone and for those with poorly demonstrated lesions. Compression can cause difficulty in precisely determining the location of a lesion because it is not possible to center the nipple in the manner described above and because breast anatomy is distorted. Compression has, however, contributed valuable information in the diagnosis of some solid lesions, giving better definition of border characteristics and internal echo content (see Figures 19 and 20). The value of compression is being studied further in the SSBDC. The symptomatology of patients referred to the SSDBC for assessment of a breast problem is given in Table 2.

TABLE 2. Symptomatology of Referred Patients

Symptom	Percent of Clinic Population
Lump	38.0*
Pain	24.0
Lumpy	8.0
Nple disch, invsn	
Itchy, ulcerated	8.0
Thickening	7.0
Enlargement	4.0
Mammographic abnormality	3.0
Risk factors	3.0
Cancerphobia	2.0
None	2.0
Previous mastectomy	0.5
Skin change	0.5
	100.0

* 4% of these patients had cancer.

INTERPRETATION OF SONOGRAMS

For the purpose of this chapter, we will assume that mammography is used in the diagnosis of breast cancer. The complementary role of sonography in breast cancer will be illustrated, with emphasis on those lesions with equivocal clinical or mammographic findings. We do not waste manpower, time and money performing sonography on a fatty breast in which a carcinoma is readily visualized mammographically but instead concentrate on the breast with mammographic densities or clinical thickenings, the nature of which is uncertain.

The signs sonographically indicative of malignancy, in order of importance, are as follows:

a) disturbance of skin line,
b) disturbance of architecture,
c) appearance of a mass,
d) changes in posterior detail on simple scan, and
e) changes in surrounding breast tissue.

Skin Line

With the breast dependent in the waterbath we have found that the skin line is a very sensitive indicator of underlying pathology. *Skin dimpling* may be the only evidence of underlying malignancy, which was the case with the 43-year-old patient whose sonograms are presented in Figure 1. There is no obvious sonographic mass within the breast tissue, despite the extensive area of skin involvement. Neither was this involvement seen clinically as a skin dimple. Mammography showed marked dysplastic changes with consequent dim-

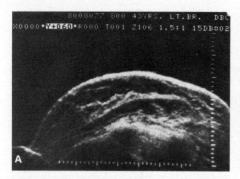 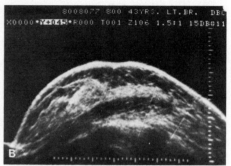

Figure 1. (*A*) Skin flattening is noted 6 cm above nipple in this 43-year-old woman who had an 8-month history of left breast thickening. (*B*) 4.5 cm above the nipple the flattening becomes a definite skin dimple. No underlying mass is visualized in the echogram. Mammography showed marked dysplasia, but no discrete mass was seen. Biopsy proved an infiltrating duct carcinoma.

inution of diagnostic ability, and no mass or microcalcification was seen. Clinically, the patient was thought to have benign thickening, but invasive carcinoma was proved at biopsy.

A careful history is important to the diagnosis, as is seen in the case of the 41-year-old woman whose sonograms are shown in Figure 2. The skin dimple (Figure 2A), seen some distance away from the cancer mass (Figure 2B), is due to scarring from previous biopsy 2 cm below nipple level. The mass lesion, which proved to be an infiltrating duct carcinoma, is 2 cm above the nipple and 4 cm from the skin dimple. Clinically and mammographically, the lesion was diagnosed as a fibroadenoma. *Flattening* may be subtle, as is illustrated

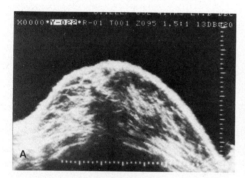 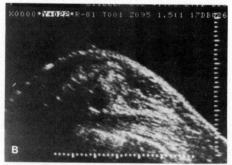

Figure 2. (*A*) A well-marked skin dimple is seen in this compound scan 22 mm below nipple level in the medial quadrant of the left breast. No underlying pathology is evident. Careful history showed the dimple to be due to scarring from previous biopsy. (*B*) A simple scan of the same breast 22 mm above nipple level in the midline clearly shows a partly irregular area of low-level echoes with a sharp posterior border that gives the sonographic appearance of a benign tumor. A solid lesion in a 41-year-old, however, is always suspicious, and biopsy was recommended. The surgeon felt the lesion was benign. Mammography demonstrated a possible cyst. Biopsy proved an infiltrating intraduct lesion. None of 31 nodes removed were metastatic.

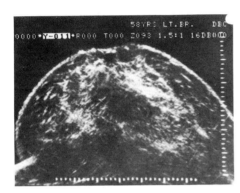

Figure 3. A compound scan echogram with skin flattening and slight dimpling 11 mm below nipple level in the midline. No underlying mass is visualized, and the breast is composed largely of fat. Mammography in this 58-year-old asymptomatic woman demonstrated a well-defined 8-mm mass associated with apparently benign calcification thought to be a duct papilloma. The lesion was not palpable, but biopsy proved the presence of a small, localized infiltrating ductal carcinoma. The axillary nodes were negative.

in Figure 3. This patient, aged 58 years, was referred to us for a mammographic follow-up of a small retroareolar mass associated with coarse calcification, thought to be benign. The presence of central flattening below the nipple in the midline raised the suspicion of the reporting physician and biopsy was recommended. The lesion proved to be an 8-mm intraduct carcinoma.

Clinically, occult carcinomata characterized by mammographic microcalcifications are not ultrasonographically demonstrated as abnormalities within the breast. However, sonographic skin changes have been seen in some of these tumors, which, although impalpable, may be surprisingly extensive. It is gratifying when a clinically unsuspected cancer is defined as an obvious and suspicious lesion on sonography, usually in an area of mammographic density in which no cancer is seen (see Figure 15).

Flattening may be gross and obvious, as is shown in Figure 4A. This patient suffered clinical Paget's disease of the nipple, but no discrete clinical abnormality had been found within the breast tissue. Extensive skin thickening and

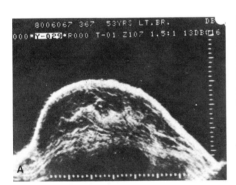
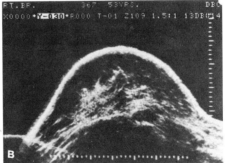

Figure 4. (A) Compound scan 2.9 cm below the left nipple demonstrating gross skin flattening and thickening. No obvious mass or other abnormality is seen within the parenchyma. Compare with B. (B) Compound scan 3.0 cm below the right nipple showing normal skin outline and thickness. This 53-year-old patient had clinically obvious Paget's disease of the left nipple. Mammography demonstrates innumerable, widespread microcalcifications in the left lower breast, but no abnormality was palpable. Biopsy proved extensive intraduct and infiltrating duct carcinoma in association with Paget's disease. Axillary nodes were negative.

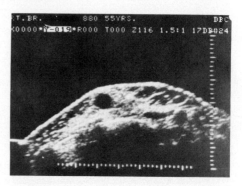

Figure 5. Compound scan 1.9 cm below the nipple shows a skin protrusion overlying a very well-defined, echo-free lesion with enhancement of posterior detail, which was more marked on simple scan. Histology showed a medullary carcinoma with central necrosis at the margins of which a well-differentiated infiltrating lobular carcinoma was described.

flattening were noted well below the nipple (compare this tissue with that from approximately the same level in the unaffected breast [Figure 4B]). Mammography in this patient demonstrated innumerable microcalcifications typical of extensive intraduct carcinoma, which was confirmed by biopsy. Despite the skin involvement and apparent size of the lesion, axillary nodes were histologically negative.

Protrusion may be slight, as is illustrated by the sonogram (Figure 5) of a medullary carcinoma found in a 55-year-old woman whose other breast had been removed for intraduct carcinoma 9 years before.

Gross protrusion is seen in the large 5.5-cm inflammatory mass with a centrally located, 2.5-cm, poorly differentiated adenocarcinoma depicted in Figure 6. The inflammatory reaction in this patient gave the clinical impression of abscess, and there was a history of recent skin breakdown with discharge of pus. Inflammatory lesions have proved to be the most difficult to diagnose clinically, mammographically and ultrasonically. The obvious problem with management of inflammatory lesions is that surgical interference is contraindicated during the acute diffuse stage because of the possibility of spread of infection to other parts of the breast or body. Very careful follow-up is essential in patients whose apparent breast mass decreases with antibiotic therapy. A carcinoma may underly the inflammation, as was found in this patient as well as in two others we have examined.

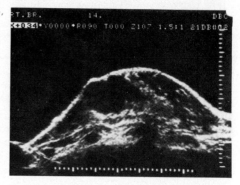

Figure 6. Compound scan of a large, almost echo-free area with marked protrusion of the overlying skin. There is compression of surrounding tissue and apparent distortion of pectoral fascia. The patient, aged 42, had a 3-week history of right breast lump and a 1-week history of pain after trauma. Clinically, the lesion was inflammatory and had broken through the skin with discharge of inflammatory material 2 weeks before the clinic visit. Mammography showed the mass to be dense and nonspecific. Histology showed a 6-cm inflammatory lesion within which a 2.5-cm infiltrating ductal carcinoma was identified.

Skin thickening and skin edema also are seen in inflammatory processes, and the differential diagnosis in these cases is often difficult. Postoperative scarring may cause skin retraction and thickening (Figure 7A), and these factors must be noted by the sonographer for the guidance of the reading physician because such scarring, with or without disruption of architecture, may mimic cancer. Skin lesions must also be recorded.

In our experience with 150 proven cancers examined sonographically, the skin line is the most consistent and often the only positive evidence of malignancy. In many cases, and almost always in the fatty breast, no other sonographic abnormality is detected because the acoustic properties of fat resemble those of cellular tumors. Fortunately, in these patients mammography usually is diagnostic (Table 1).

Disturbance of Architecture

Disturbance of architecture may be minimal, as is shown in Figure 8. Some protrusion of the skin medial to the nipple, under which is a subtle break in glandular architecture, is seen in this and other frames. Clinically, the mass was visible and obviously malignant. The overlying skin was dimpled, but mammography was nonspecific and sonography raised the suspicion in this patient. A 3-cm infiltrating duct carcinoma was demonstrated by biopsy.

Straightening of Cooper's ligaments is seen in Figures 9, 10A and 11A, all associated with underlying masses. In Figure 12A an area of low-level echoes 17 mm lateral to the nipple and distortion of surrounding fibrous tissue and ligaments are seen. In Figure 12B, 1.3 cm more medial the distortion of Coop-

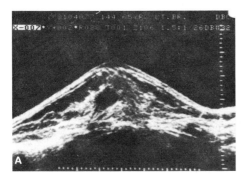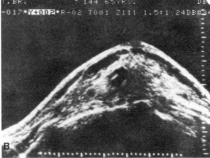

Figure 7. (A) Compound sagittal scan 7 mm medial to the left nipple in this 65-year-old patient clearly demonstrated gross skin thickening and edema. Within the parenchyma, there is an apparent echo-free area with irregular but not jagged margins. Skin thickening added to the suspicion in this lesion. Several foci of carcinoma were proven by biopsy. (B) Compound transverse scan of the right breast in the same patient show mixed pathology. The larger lesion with the bright echo is a fibroadenoma with macrocalcification. The smaller area of low-level echoes 1-cm lateral to the first mass had, in other frames, irregular borders and carcinoma was diagnosed. Adenocarcinoma of the left axillary lymph node had been diagnosed elsewhere, but despite the extent of the malignancy in both breasts found during our investigation, no further axillary nodes showed metastatic disease.

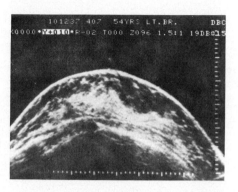

Figure 8. Compound sagittal scan in a 54-year-old woman shows a subtle disturbance of architecture and parenchymal outline, with a suggestion of skin protrusion overlying the area. Mammography showed equivocal calcifications in this clinically malignant lesion.

er's ligaments is strikingly obvious, and the underlying carcinoma is no longer visualized.

An illustration of the scirrhous component of the fibrous reaction to an underlying carcinoma is seen in Figure 13. This 40-year-old woman presented with a 2.5-cm clinically diagnosed malignant tumor, which, because of its position, tethered to the pectoral fascia, was not well demonstrated by film mammography or xeromammography. Ultrasonography not only illustrates the irregular area of low-level echoes and disruption of pectoral fascia at the site of the cancer, but the fibrous strands in this tubular carcinoma are clearly seen extending throughout the breast tissue and pulling in the skin up to 5 cm from the tumor on the opposite side of the nipple.

Disruption of glandular tissue is best seen in the dense breast, and in Figure 14 an irregular area of low-level echoes is immediately obvious in the otherwise homogeneous high-level echoes of active dysplastic breast tissue. Clinically, this patient, aged 55 years, was thought to have a fibroadenoma. Mammography showed dysplasia but no mass was visualized.

Similar architectural, skin, and fibrous tissue changes may be seen in postbiopsy scarring, fat necrosis, and in patients who have undergone reduction mammoplasty. Such factors are confirmed by history and clinical observation.

Definition of a Mass

A true solid or cystic mass is usually seen on both the transerve and sagittal sections and should be followed in 1-mm increments along its boundaries to

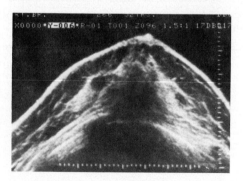

Figure 9. Compound sagittal scan in this 52-year-woman shows straightened Cooper's ligaments coming from an irregular area of low-level echoes. As in the scan pictured in Figure 8, there is a suggestion of skin protrusion. Mammography showed marked dysplasia but no mass. The lesion was clinically suspicious. Biopsy showed infiltrating duct carcinoma. Axillary nodes were negative.

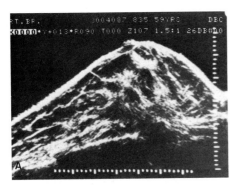
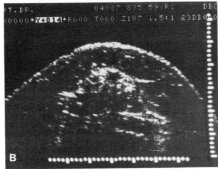

Figure 10. (A) Compound transverse scan in this 59-year-old woman shows a thickened and straightened Cooper's ligament arising from an irregular area of very low-level echoes with some surrounding fibrous reaction. (B) On rotation of the gantry through 90°, the simple scan shows an irregular, almost echo-free area with refractive shadowing of posterior detail, giving most of the sonographic signs of malignancy. Clinically, the patient was thought to have Paget's disease of the nipple. Mammography detected a carcinoma within the breast that was not palpable, the lesion seen on sonography. The biopsy showed primary infiltrating duct carcinoma extending into nipple. Axillary nodes were negative.

explore the nature of its surface and internal echo content. The most common "false" mass is due to entrapped fat, but careful following of the area to all its boundaries usually shows merging into other areas of fat. Figure 7A demonstrates an irregular area containing few, if any echoes which, when combined with gross edema of overlying skin and refractive shadowing seen in other views, was interpreted as suspicious of malignancy. Figure 7B shows multiple pathology. The more central, larger lesion being a fibroadenoma associated with macrocalcification, is seen here as the bright white echo. Just lateral to this, the irregular area of low-level echoes was diagnosed as a carcinoma ul-

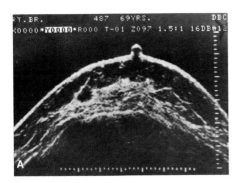
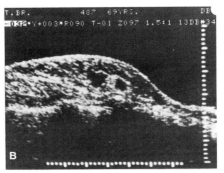

Figure 11. (A) Compound sagittal scan in a 69-year-old patient shows an irregular area of low-level echoes with a straightened Cooper's ligament. (B) Simple scan on rotation through the lesion shows a jagged boundary, some enhancement of posterior detail and surrounding fibrous reaction. Mammography showed an atypical, slightly irregular mass thought to be probably benign on clinical examination. Biopsy proved a 1.6-cm anaplastic carcinoma. Axillary nodes were negative.

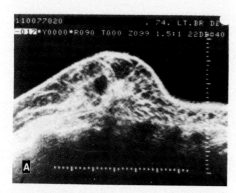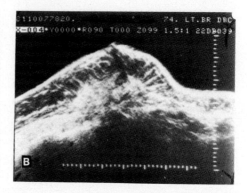

Figure 12. (*A*) Compound sagittal scan in a patient, aged 74, shows a nonspecific area of very low-level echoes above the nipple with marked fibrosis below the mass. (*B*) Straightening and distortion of Cooper's ligaments is well demonstrated below the nipple in this compound scan. Mammography and clinical examination suggested a malignant lesion. Biopsy proved anaplastic carcinoma.

trasonically. The 65-year-old patient presented with a single, large left axillary node containing carcinoma "query breast" in origin. Bilateral carcinoma was confirmed by biopsy, with no further axillary node involvement. Figure 15A demonstrates a 5-mm carcinoma in a 43-year-old woman seen in the transverse view as an irregular area of low-level echoes 5 cm above nipple level just lateral to the midline. On rotation through 90°, the area is displayed even more obviously (Figure 15B) as a very irregular area of low-level echoes, which is highly indicative of carcinoma. The clinical impression was of a vague thickening and mammography was suspicious but inconclusive.

In Figure 10A an area of low-level echoes is seen 14-mm above nipple level. Rotation of the gantry through 90° gives the image shown in Figure 10B. Suspicion is increased by the surrounding fibrous reaction and straightened Cooper's ligament, which is well demonstrated.

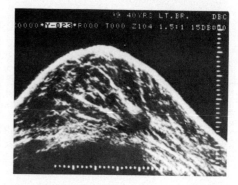

Figure 13. Compound transverse scan in a woman, aged 40, with a clinically suspicious mass shows an irregular area of low-level echoes with a marked scirrhous component and fibrous strands extending across the breast to the skin on other side of the nipple. The carcinoma was deeply located on pectoral fascia and consequently not well displayed by mammography. Biopsy proved a 1-cm, largely tubular carcinoma. One axillary node was positive.

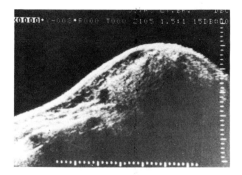

Figure 14. Compound sagittal scan in a 55-year-old woman with a clinical fibroadenoma showed a jagged, almost anechoic area in the upper part of the breast that was highly indicative of carcinoma. Mammography was negative due to marked dysplasia. Biopsy proved an 8-mm intraduct carcinoma. Axillary nodes were histologically negative.

Nature of Mass Boundary

Irregular or jagged borders and low-level echo content are seen in most malignant lesions (see descriptions above and Figures 11B, 14 and 15B). Localized areas of active dysplasia show irregular boundaries and low-level echo content and only extensive experience and confidence in the testing situation together with mammographic correlation will result in accurate diagnosis. Smooth, well-defined borders are seen in cysts, fibroadenomata, lipomata, and other less-common benign lesions. Smooth borders in malignant lesions are seen in the medullary carcinoma shown in Figure 5. Ultrasonically, this lesion was indistinguishable from a cyst, but suspicion was aroused by the obvious skin protrusion over the tumor.

Both benign and malignant lesions may appear lobulated, as is seen in the mixed pathology tumor shown in Figure 6. This lobulated lesion is a 2.5-cm carcinoma within a 5-cm inflammatory mass.

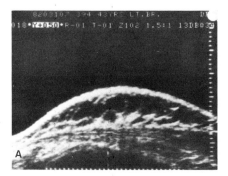
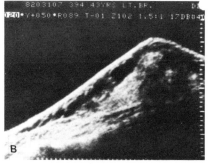

Figure 15. (A) Compound transverse scan in a 43-year-old woman shows a jagged collection of low-level echoes that is suspicious in outline. (B) On rotation into the sagittal plane, the suspicious mass is even better demonstrated. Mammography was negative but showed dysplasia. The clinical examination suggested a benign lesion. Biopsy proved a 5-mm infiltrating duct carcinoma. Axillary nodes were histologically negative.

Nature of Internal Echoes

A typical intraduct carcinoma contains low-level echoes within a jagged or irregular border, and most of the lesions illustrated in this chapter show one or both of these features. Absence of internal echoes within a mass at relatively high gain settings is typical of a cyst. Figure 5 shows a typical medullary carcinoma, and because this mass is echo free it could be confused with a cyst. Homogeneous medium-level echoes within a well-defined border are typical of a fibroadenoma but may also be seen in a debris-filled abscess and in some cysts with particulate matter suspended within the cyst fluid.

Because of the similar echo content in fat and cellular cancers, fatty entrapment is the most common "false" tumor. Well-defined areas of fat may be differentiated from true tumors by following the "lesion" in 1- to 2-mm increments around the borders to determine size and shape. An area of fat often merges into other areas and is not usually seen in right-angled views of the "lesion."

A solid tumor with well-defined but angular borders is seen in Figure 16. This 39-year-old woman had a lesion described clinically and mammographically as a fibroadenoma. Sonography demonstrated a mass with rather pointed corners, and refractive shadowing added to the suspicion that it was malignant. An 18-mm infiltrating duct carcinoma was proved by biopsy.

Nature of Surrounding Tissue

Compression of surrounding tissue by a space-occupying lesion is more commonly present in benign than in malignant tumors, and is seen in chronic abscesses and some thick-walled cysts. However, in some cancers, a dense fibrotic reaction is produced and Cooper's ligaments may be distorted (Figure 13).

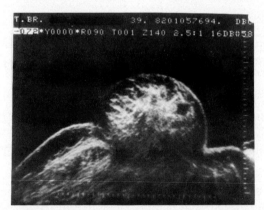

Figure 16. A 39-year-old woman was referred to us with a mass thought to be a fibroadenoma. Mammography showed a fairly well-defined mass. This compound sagittal sonogram shows a mass with irregular outline. Biopsy proved a 1.8-cm infiltrating duct carcinoma.

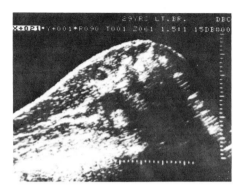

Figure 17. Simple sagittal sonogram in a woman, aged 29, with a clinically suspicious mass above the nipple shows an area of low-level echoes with distinct refractive shadowing. Mammography showed a non-specific increase in density within a dysplastic lobule. Biopsy proved an infiltrating ductal carcinoma. Axillary nodes were negative.

Nature of Posterior Beam

Single transducer scans are recorded from various angles through areas of suspicion.

In our experience with more than 150 proven cancers, *central shadowing* of posterior detail has not been a reliable indicator of malignancy. Central shadowing of posterior detail is seen consistently in areas of active dysplasia as well as behind the nipple, behind scars, and behind dense ridges of fibrous tissue.

Refractive or peripheral shadowing coming from the edges of the lesion has been seen in proven fibroadenomata and in some carcinomata, as in the 29-year-old woman whose sonogram is shown in Figure 17. Clinically, the lesion was suspicious for malignant, but mammography was nonspecific even though the breast tissue was not particularly dysplastic.

Although *enhancement* of posterior detail on simple scanning is the typical property of a cystic lesion, medullary carcinomata may also have this property, as is illustrated in Figure 5.

General Nature of Breast Tissue

In some larger and in all inflammatory carcinomata, generalized edema of breast tissue is ultrasonically obvious, especially when compared with the unaffected breast. This edema usually is associated with generalized skin thickening, and the skin may have a double-layered appearance, as shown in Figure 7a. The 38-year-old patient whose sonogram is shown in Figure 18, was referred to us with a 3-year history of increasing left nipple inversion and enlargement of the left breast. The patient had undergone a right mastectomy for breast cancer 3 years previously. The clinical picture of advanced carcinoma was confirmed by mammography, which showed skin thickening and a 4-cm spiculated mass medial to the left nipple. Sonographically, not only was the nipple inverted, but the skin was thickened and edematous. The breast tissue showed almost homogeneous high-level echoes, which we have come to associate with generalized edema of the breast. The differentiation between inflammatory carcinoma and simple inflammatory lesion is extremely difficult using any modality and very careful follow-up of all such cases is essential.

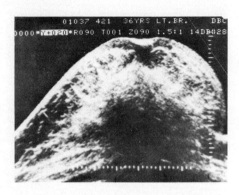

Figure 18. This compound transverse scan in a 36-year-old woman demonstrates nipple inversion, skin thickening and generalized edema of breast tissue. No discrete mass is visualized. Clinically, a large mass was felt above the nipple, and mammography demonstrated a scirrhous tumor. Biopsy proved an 8-cm infiltrating duct carcinoma.

Usefulness of Compression

In a 37-year-old woman who presented with a right breast lump, the clinical findings were equivocal. Mammography showed a suspicious lesion associated with faint microcalcifications. Compound sonographic scans of the uncompressed breast (Figure 19A), showed a nonspecific area of medium-level echoes similar to the surrounding areas of fat. No shadowing of posterior detail was seen on simple scan. When the breast was compressed against the chest wall (Figure 19B), the fat was compressed into insignificance but the tumor is clearly demonstrated. Biopsy proved a 1-cm mucoid carcinoma.

A 48-year-old woman came to us with a 3-week history of right breast lump. The lesion felt suspicious but mammography showed dense dysplasia and no mass was visualized. Sonography of the uncompressed breast (Figure 20A) produced a strong echo below the nipple. Such an echo usually is regarded as due to fibrous tissue. The surrounding low-level echoes were nonspecific. On compression of the breast against the chest wall (Figure 20B), the strong echo of fibrous content was seen to be surrounded by a large area of low-level echoes with irregular lobulated margins, the nature of which was uncertain sono-

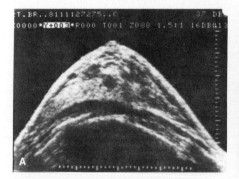
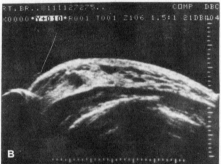

Figure 19. (A) Uncompressed compound transverse sonogram in a woman, aged 37, with an equivocal clinical mass suggests an area of low-level echoes in the midline of the breast behind the nipple. Mammography demonstrated a mass with microcalcifications. (B) On compression, the mass appears larger (fat, when compressed, usually spreads and appears smaller) and is better defined. Biopsy proved a 1-cm mucoid carcinoma. Axillary nodes were histologically negative.

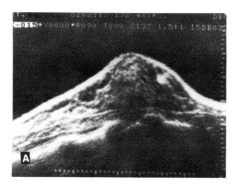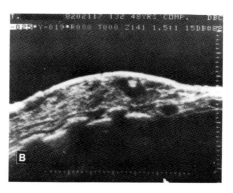

Figure 20. (A) Compound sagittal scan in a 48-year-old patient shows a mass of fibrous tissue, seen as bright echoes below the nipple, the nature of which was uncertain sonographically. Clinically, a hard mass suggested malignant disease. Mammography showed marked dysplasia in the retroareolar region, with no obvious mass or other abnormality. (B) Compound sagittal sonogram of the same patient with the breast compressed shows the fibrous tissue, but it is now seen to be surrounded by a fairly well-defined area of suspicious low-level echoes. A very aggressive 2-cm infiltrating ductal carcinoma was proven at biopsy. One axillary node was histologically positive.

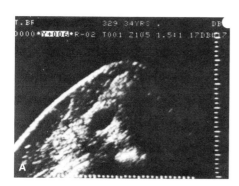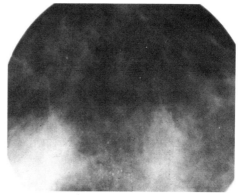

Figure 21. (A) Simple transverse sonogram in a patient, aged 34, who presented with pain illustrates a simple cystic lesion that had been palpated by the Clinic surgeons. (B) The mammogram of the same patient shows the two simple cystic lesions seen on echography and also grouped microcalcifications between the cysts. Histological examination proved this impalpable calcified area to be intraductal carcinoma with early encephaloid carcinoma. This case emphasizes the importance of using the complementary tests of mammography and sonography in the investigation of patients with breast symptoms.

105

TABLE 3.   Results of Breast Echography is 14 Patients with Proven Breast Cancer That Was Not Palpated

Number of Patients	Sonography			Total
	Positive	Suspicious	Negative	
14	7 (50%)	4 (28%)	3 (21%)	14

graphically but which was considered suspicious. Biopsy proved an extensive and very aggressive cellular adenocarcinoma.

Warning

Sonography may demonstrate a benign lesion, which may also be palpable, but it may miss small carcinomata that can be detected mammographically. A 34-year-old woman presented with bilateral breast pain and a recent lump in her right breast. Sonography correctly demonstrated the simple cysts within the breast (Figure 21A), but did not reveal the impalpable carcinoma characterized by the mammographic calcifications seen between the cysts in Figure 21B.

SONOGRAPHY COMPARED WITH SURGICAL OPINION IN 190 CASES OF BREAST CANCER

In patients described by the examining surgeon as normal or as having diffuse benign disease, that is, those in whom no breast tumor was felt, we were able to ultrasonographically demonstrate a solid lesion or an area of suspicion in 11 of 14 cases (Table 3). A tumor may not only be impalpable because it consists of microcalcifications or because it is too small but also because it may be deeply located or lie within very active breast tissue. The interpreting physician can report only on those images supplied to him by his technician. As in mammography, examination of the patient by the technician performing the test is essential if palpable lesions are to be well demonstrated (Tables 4 and 5). Of 17 palpable lesions that were diagnosed as probably benign by the

TABLE 4.   Results of Breast Echography in 19 Patients with Proven Breast Cancer That the Examining Surgeon Had Diagnosed as a Benign Mass

Number of Patients	Sonography			Total
	Positive	Suspicious	Negative	
19	10 53%	0	9 (47%)	19

TABLE 5. Results of Breast Echography in 7 Patients with Proven Breast Cancer That the Examining Surgeon Had Diagnosed as a "Probably Benign" Mass

Number of Patients	Sonography			Total
	Positive	Suspicious	Negative	
17	10 (59%)	3 (18%)	4 (23%)	17

examining surgeon and that histologically were found to be malignant, 13 were ultrasonographically diagnosed as malignant or suspicious (Table 5).

Of the remainder of the 186 patients with proven breast cancer who were examined by sonography, 136 (72%) were reported as having suspicious or frankly malignant lesions on clinical examination. Ultrasonography was reported as positive or suspicious in 80%.

An advantage of sonography lies in its ability to reduce the number of biopsies performed to check the clinical or mammographic diagnosis of a lesion. Simple cysts that the surgeon has called suspicious on clinical grounds have been proven sonographically in many patients. This misdiagnosis is usually due to active dysplasia surrounding the cysts, causing the whole area to feel irregular and therefore suspicious. The ability of sonography to correctly sort mamographically and clinically diagnosed masses into cystic or solid, of course, permits appropriate management.

CONCLUSION

The value of ultrasonography in the diagnosis of breast cancer has been discussed in this chapter. Using the sonographic techniques described, we have detected cancers as small as 5 mm in glandular breast tissue. Conversely, we have been unable to demonstrate cancers as large as 3 cm in atrophic fatty breasts. For this reason, sonography is not used as a stand-alone test in patients with breast symptoms who are older than about 25 years, and correlation with recent and adequate film-screen mammography is routine in our clinic. Nevertheless, the value of sonography in the investigation of breast disease is now firmly established.

ACKNOWLEDGMENTS

The author wishes to thank the trustees of the A. W. Tyree Foundation for the establishment of this non-profit-making Diagnostic Clinic; sonographers Jane Kotevich, Jan Waddington and Margaret Tabrett for the production of sonograms of excellent quality and for their help in writing this chapter; Paula Bosman for her voluntary work in following up clinic patients; and Dr. Raymond Healey and Elizabeth Croll for their help in data entry and correlation of results.

8

HEPATOCELLULAR CARCINOMA: DIAGNOSIS BY REAL-TIME ULTRASONOGRAPHY

Yutaka Atomi

Sumio Inoue

Nobuhiro Kawano

Yasuhiko Morioka

Although hepatocellular carcinoma (HCC) is rare in the western world, it is one of the most common causes of death by malignant neoplasm in Japan. For this reason the clinicians in this country have considerable interest in the diagnostic aspects of this disease. If HCC is detected early and found to be resectable, it may be cured by surgery. Unfortunately, the operative results from many institutes are not encouraging (1, 2).

Ultrasonography has been one of the major advances in the diagnostic imaging of the liver, not only because it is noninvasive but also because it provides true cross-sectional images (3, 4). With the bistable equipment, evaluation of liver size and contour is relatively accurate (5), but it is not possible to assess the internal architecture of the liver (5, 6). The detection of focal lesions of the liver has been greatly advanced by the advent of gray scale echography (7–13). The weak echoes of normal liver parenchyma can be clearly demonstrated and slight changes in its echo-pattern detected. With modern equipment the accuracy of detecting HCC is approaching 90%. The skill of the ultrasonographer is very crucial to the accuracy and validity of the examination.

Real-time equipment is one of the recent technological advances in diagnostic ultrasonography (4). Although it was originally developed for cardiac imaging, real-time studies have become widely accepted for imaging other parts of the body as well (14). The principal advantage of using real-time ultrasound in abdominal imaging is that it provides greater flexibility and maneuverability compared with conventional articulated-arm scanners (14).

Many reports have been published describing the value and role of gray scale ultrasonography (7–12, 15), but, to date, only a few reports mention the

108

application of real-time ultrasonography in the diagnosis of hepatic diseases, especially of HCC.

In this chapter we will discuss the diagnostic accuracy of real-time ultrasound in HCC and describe the correlations with histologic type, angiographic vascularity and ultrasonic examinations.

CLINICAL MATERIALS AND METHODS

Our series consists of 28 patients (26 men and 2 women, aged 31 to 72) with histologically proved HCC who were examined consecutively during 4 years by real-time ultrasonography.

Selective angiographic examinations of the liver also were performed and the findings were compared with the results of the ultrasonic examination of 27 patients. Computed tomographic (CT) examinations were performed in all cases.

The examinations were performed with commercially available linear-array real-time ultrasound equipment (Toshiba SAL 10-A, 30-A and Yokokawa RT 100F). Both 2.24- and 3.5-MHz transducers were used. Most of studies were recorded with a Polaroid camera; a few were recorded with a single-format camera (Fuji FSC1010).

ACCURACY OF REAL-TIME
ULTRASONOGRAPHY IN DETECTION OF HCC

Using real-time ultrasound, we were able to correctly detect the lesion in 27 of 28 patients (97%). This result was compatible with those of angiography (96%) and of computed tomography (93%).

Ten patients had multiple lesions, while 18 had solitary lesions. The smallest solitary HCC lesion detected was 2 cm in its greatest diameter. Solitary 1-cm HCC lesions were not demonstrated. This is in contrast to patients with multiple lesions in whom HCC lesions 1 cm in diameter could be clearly demonstrated.

MACROSCOPIC FINDINGS OF HCC AND
ULTRASONOGRAPHIC PATTERNS

HCC may be classified into (a) nodular, (b) massive and (c) diffuse types on the basis of the macroscopic findings of Eggel (16). This classification correlates well with the ultrasonographic findings in that all nodular types showed discrete echographic patterns (Figure 1), while all massive types showed massive patterns (Figure 2). In our series no diffuse-type hepatoma was encountered. We classified the 28 cases of HCC according to the number of tumors, configuration and internal ultrasonic patterns as given in Table 1. With regard to internal echo patterns, of five cases of small HCC (less than 2 cm) four showed a low echo pattern (Figure 1A and B), while high and mixed patterns were frequently seen in lesions greater than 2 cm (Table 1; Figure 3A and B). Of

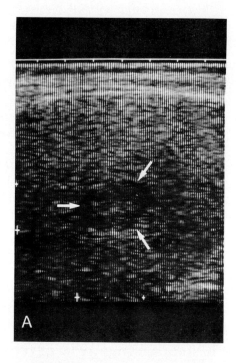

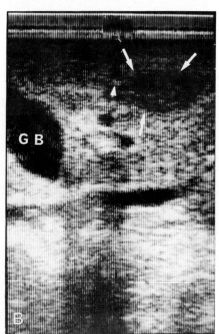

Figure 1. Hepatoma. (*A*) Right subcostal echogram displaying hypoechoic tumor (arrows). (*B*) This tumor was confirmed to be HCC by aspiration biopsy under ultrasonographic imaging. Arrows, hepatoma; arrowhead, needle tip; GB, gallbladder.

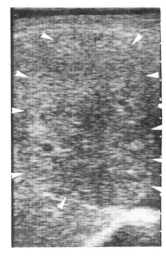

Figure 2. Hepatoma. Subcostal echogram displaying massive-type hepatoma (arrowheads).

23 patients showing high or mixed echo patterns, 20 had necrosis and/or bleeding within the tumors (Table 2; Figure 4A and B). In contrast, none of the five cases classified as low internal echo type exhibited necrosis and/or bleeding. It is generally accepted that the echoes returned to the transducer are due to a scattering process within tissue. Small metastatic lesions may be less echogenic, and as lesions become larger they can display internal echoes from

TABLE 1. Ultrasonographic Patterns of HCC

Diameter of Tumor	Nodular Solitary	Multiple	Massive	Diffuse
<2 cm	1	4	0	0
2–5 cm	7	5	0	0
≥5 cm	4	1	6	0

TABLE 1. (Continued)

Diameter of Tumor	Internal Echo			Halo (capsule)	Lobular
	Low	High	Mixed		
<2 cm	4	1	0	0	0
2–5 cm	1	7	4	4 (5)	3
≥5 cm	0	6	5	2 (4)	2

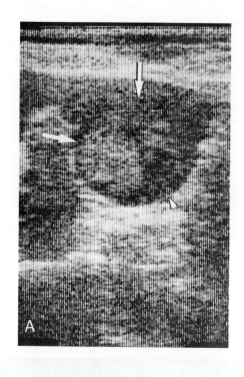

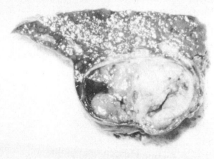

Figure 3. Hepatoma. (*A*) Transverse echogram displaying partially hyperechoic (arrows) and partially hypoechoic (arrowhead) tumor. This belongs to nodular, mixed and lobular type. (*B*) Surgical specimen is well correlated to ultrasonographic findings.

TABLE 2. Ultrasonographic Pattern and Macroscopic Necrosis and/or Bleeding

		Low	High	Mixed
Necrosis and/or Bleeding	(+)	0	12	8
	(−)	5	0	0

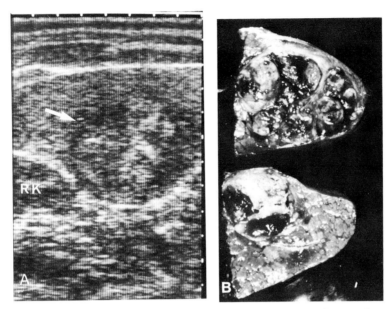

Figure 4. Hepatoma. (*A*) Right oblique echogram displaying mixed tumor (arrow). RK, right kidney. (*B*) Surgical specimen showing necrosis and bleeding within the hepatoma.

organization degeneration or necrosis. Nine cases had fibrous pseudocapsule macroscopically. Six of these showed a halo with an echogenic center and a surrounding area that was relatively sonolucent (Figure 5). Haloes, however, were occasionally seen in metastatic liver tumors (7). We could not find a specific ultrasonic pattern of HCC to differentiate them from metastatic liver

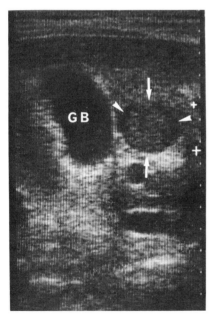

Figure 5. Hepatoma. Subcostal echogram displaying small hepatoma (arrows) with halo (arrowheads). GB, gallbladder.

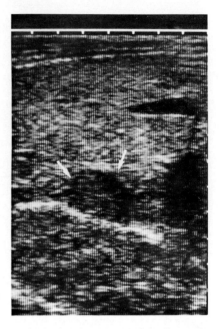

Figure 6. Metastatic liver tumor. Tumor is hypoechoic (arrows). Primary site was colon.

tumor or other intrahepatic neoplasms (Figure 6). Five cases of HCC showed a fine lobular pattern, corresponding to the macroscopic lobular pattern (Figure 3A). This pattern was not seen in most of the metastatic tumors, and we think that this pattern could be specific to HCC.

ANGIOGRAPHIC CORRELATION (TABLE 3)

The ultrasound patterns were compared with the degree of vascularity of the tumors in all 27 patients who underwent hepatic angiography. Only two cases showed hypovascular or avascular findings. One was a massive echogenic type, the other a massive mixed type. No definite association between vascularity and ultrasound pattern could be established.

CIRRHOSIS AND ULTRASONOGRAPHIC PATTERNS (TABLE 4)

Although it has been suggested (17) that cirrhosis affects the ultrasonic pattern of HCC, no definite association between cirrhosis and ultrasound pattern could be established in our series.

TABLE 3. Angiographic Vascularity and Ultrasonographic Patterns

Angiography		Ultrasonographic Patterns
Hypervascular	25	
Hypovascular	1	Massive echogenic
Avascular	1	Massive mixed

TABLE 4.   Ultrasonographic Pattern and Liver Cirrhosis (LC)

	Ultrasonographic Pattern				
	Low	High	Mixed	(Lobular)	Halo
LC (+)	5	12	6	5	5
LC (−)	0	2	3	0	1

These findings suggest that it is extremely difficult to ultrasonically differentiate HCC from other intrahepatic tumors, except in a few cases showing the fine lobular pattern.

ASSOCIATED FINDINGS IN ULTRASONOGRAPHY OF HCC

Cirrhosis

Inasmuch as in approximately 80% of cases HCC are associated with cirrhosis, it is important to be able to differentiate these conditions.

The internal echoes of the liver are more numerous and intense in cirrhosis, but this also is seen in other diffuse parenchymal liver diseases (18, 19). Caudate lobe hypertrophy is frequently observed in cirrhotic patients (20). The penetration of the sound beam is decreased and the size of the lesion and the branches of the portal vein become less apparent in advanced stages (19). Demonstration of splenomegaly, ascites and dilated umbilical vein (21) is also helpful in confirming cirrhosis. Taking all of these findings into account, it is generally not difficult to make the diagnosis of advanced stage cirrhosis in most cases. In our series, there were 23 cases (82%) of cirrhosis, half of which were correctly diagnosed ultrasonically.

Tumor Thrombi in Portal or Hepatic Vein

Tumor thrombi frequently are seen in the portal and hepatic veins as well as the inferior vena cava of HCC patients (22) (Figure 7). Preoperative detection of these thrombi is important because it determines the surgical procedure (23). In our series, seven patients were diagnosed as having tumor thrombi in the portal or hepatic vein, as is shown in Table 5. Real-time ultrasonography and CT were very useful in the detection of these lesions (24).

TABLE 5.   Tumor Thrombi of Portal and Hepatic Veins

	Tumor Thrombi
Portal vein	5/28
Hepatic vein	2/28

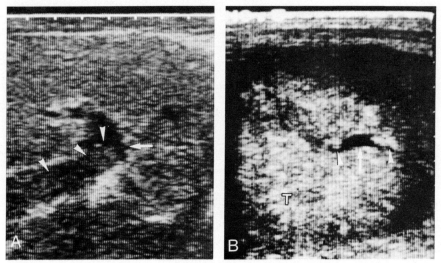

Figure 7.   (A) Tumor thrombus (arrowheads) within the portal vein (arrow). (B) Tumor thrombus (arrowheads) within middle hepatic vein (arrow). T, hepatoma.

Bile Duct Obstruction

Jaundice occurs in approximately 10–40% of patients with HCC (24). The mechanism includes associated cirrhosis, tumor infiltration into the hepatic parenchyma, lymph node compression of bile ducts and intrahepatic and extrahepatic mass compression of biliary radicles (24). An intrahepatic tumor obstructing the bile duct is a sign of possible HCC (25).

DIFFERENTIAL DIAGNOSIS OF HCC FROM OTHER SPACE-OCCUPYING LESIONS (SOL)

Metastatic Tumors

Although it has been suggested that echogenic intrahepatic tumors commonly represent metastasis from colonic or urologic primary sources (11, 26, 27), no sonographic characteristics have been described that permit the distinction of HCC from hepatic metastases. One-fifth of HCC have fine lobular patterns, which appears to be specific to HCC, and these tumors may be diagnosed by ultrasonography. Furthermore, other ultrasonographic findings, such as liver cirrhosis, portal or hepatic venous thrombosis of tumor or bile duct obstruction, facilitate the differentiation of metastases from HCC.

Hemangioma

Hemangioma, the most frequent benign tumor of the liver (28) occasionally is encountered in ultrasonographic examinations Hemangioma shows hyperechoic (Figure 8), hypoechoic and mixed patterns similar to those described for malignant tumors (29). A small hemangioma is usually demonstrated as a hyperechoic round mass. In the case of larger lesions, an appearance simulating necrotic nodules with gravity-dependent echoes within an anechoic area may be observed. Acoustic enhancement distal to the hemangioma is present in only a few cases. The absence of enhancement is presumed to be the result of multiple reflecting fibrous septa or fibrous replacement of the vascular spaces. In a few cases, a central linear septum may be clearly demonstrated by ultrasonography (29). Percutaneous biopsy for hemangioma is considered contraindicated because unexpected and excessive bleeding may result. Dynamic serial CT is very useful in such cases (30).

Liver Cell Adenoma and Focal Nodular Hyperplasia

Hepatic adenoma may be hypoechoic with or without a hyperechoic area. Similar to HCC and metastases, the ultrasonographic findings are not specific for liver cell adenoma or focal nodular hyperplasia (31, 32) (Figure 9). The absence of a known primary tumor or predisposing cause of HCC helps to distinguish these in women of childbearing age (31). Adenoma of the liver is recognized more frequently in patients with type-I glycogen storage disease (von Gierke's disease) (32). Since Kupffer cells are responsible for accumulation of Tc-Sc, theoretically only focal nodular hyperplasia should concentrate colloid. This is relatively specific for uncomplicated focal nodular hyperplasia inasmuch as a regenerating nodule of cirrhosis is the only other lesion to accumulate sulfur colloid. Because HCC may arise in a hepatic adenoma (32, 33), the changes

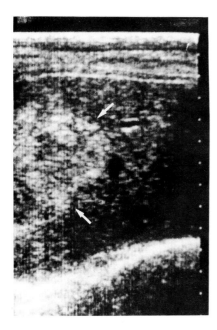

Figure 8.   Hemangioma. Right subcostal echogram displaying hyperechoic tumor (arrows).

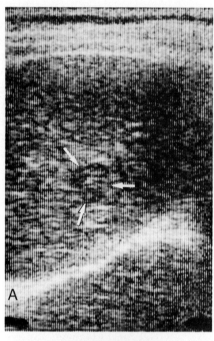

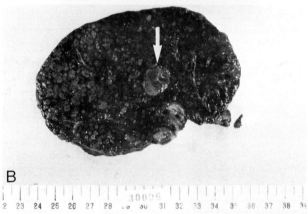

Figure 9.   Regenerative nodule. (*A*) Right subcostal echogram displaying small mixed tumor (arrows). (*B*) Autopsy specimen displaying regenerative nodule (arrow) in cirrhotic liver.

in internal echo pattern seen in rapidly growing lesions suggests a malignant change.

Abscess and Cyst

In general, it is not difficult to ultrasonographically differentiate abscesses and cysts (34) on the basis of the increased distal sonic enhancement observed in almost all cases (35) (Figure 10) and the internal echo patterns of both types

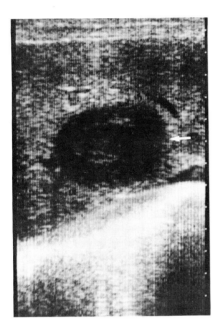

Figure 10. Abscess. Subcostal ultrasonogram displaying hypoechoic tumor (arrow).

of lesion. Some cases of abscess which change thin size and/or texture in a
short time may be diagnosed correctly by ultrasonography. Amebic abscesses
may, however, be misinterpreted as neoplasms (26, 36).

Others

Some very rare tumors, such as cystic hepatoblastoma (37) or mesenchymal
hamartoma (38), which are said to have internal septations, must be included
in the differential diagnosis of hepatic tumors. Ultrasonic pseudolesions of the
liver caused by anatomic variants or scanning artifacts no longer are a source
of interpretative error for the experienced ultrasonologist (39).

ULTRASONOGRAPHIC DIAGNOSIS OF HCC

The normal liver displays a homogeneous internal architecture with fine uniform distribution of echoes without focal defects (27). A regular pattern of
portal and hepatic veins with intervening homogeneous liver parenchyma is
the characteristic appearance of real-time scans of the liver. When smal in-
homogeneities suggesting SOL are present, they are strikingly obvious on real-
time scanning. Many ultrasonic patterns have been described for hepatic tumors (Table 6). Generally, the ultrasonographic pattern of a liver tumor consists of a mixture of two or more of the echographic patterns (7, 41).

In previous studies, the variable ultrasonographic appearance of hepatoma
has been noted. Large, irregular, highly echogenic lesions were thought to be
suggestive of HCC (12, 42). Our series indicates that it is difficult to differ-

TABLE 6. Echographic Patterns of Hepatoma

(1) *Green et al (8)*
  1. Discrete masses with increased number or strength of echoes
  2. Diffuse alteration of architecture with mixed echogenic and/or echo-free areas but without discrete masses

(2) *Kamin et al (15)*
  1. Hepatomegaly with diffuse distortion of normal internal architecture
  2. Large, focal, densely echogenic mass ranging from 2 to 12 cm
  3. Mixed pattern

(3) *Dubbins et al (17)*
  Type A: Rounded, usually well-defined lesions with predominantly low-level echoes but with several scattered internal echoes
  Type B: Predominantly echogenic lesions with poorly defined irregular margins and without definite shape
  Type C: Mixed lesions with areas of low-level echoes and area of high echogenicity. The margins of the lesions usually are well defined.
  Type D: Diffuse abnormality of liver parenchyma. Echo pattern difficult to describe in terms of relative echogenicity because of the absence of normal liver parenchyma for comparison

(4) *Broderick et al (40)*
  1. Discrete sonolucent
  2. Discrete sonodense
  3. Diffusely abnormal parenchyma without discrete lesions
  4. Normal

(5) *Hillman et al (41)*
  1. Hyperechoic
  2. Hypoechoic with central echoes

(6) *Calder (42)*
  Large, irregular, echogenic, space-occupying lesion with irregular margins

entiate HCC from other liver tumors by ultrasonography alone, with the exception of the HCC that shows a fine lobular echo pattern.

CT, hepatic angiography and percutaneous needle biopsy may be necessary for further evaluation of hepatic tumors (43).

Although the number of cases examined in our series is small, the results indicate no significant difference in sensitivity, specificity or accuracy in the detection of the liver tumors by angiography, CT and ultrasonography. Ninety-five percent of SOL in the liver were successfully detected by ultrasonography.

Although real-time instruments have been available for a number of years, it is only recently that this equipment has been applied to upper abdominal examination. The small field of view sometimes makes it difficult to identify the anatomical structure, and the experience of the ultrasonographer plays an important role. Experience indicates that ultrasonography is as capable of demonstrating anatomic structure as CT. Real-time makes it easy to direct a needle to a lesion through an optimal skin entry to establish the diagnosis of hepatic tumors, and it is likely that this equipment will replace conventional articulated-arm scanners in the near future.

REFERENCES

1. Lai CL, Lam KC, Wong KP, et al: Clinical features of hepatocellular carcinoma: review of 211 patients in Hong Kong. Cancer 47: 2746–2755, 1981.
2. Adson M: Diagnosis and surgical treatment of primary and secondary solid hepatic tumors in the adult. Surg Clin North Am 61: 181–196, 1981.
3. Smith JH, Kemey MM, Sugarbaker PH, et al: A prospective study of hepatic imaging in the detection of metastatic disease. Ann Surg 195: 486–491, 1981.
4. Cooperberg PL, Chow T, Kite V: Biparietal diameter: a comparison of real-time and conventional B-scan technique. JCU 4: 421, 1976.
5. Holm HH: Ultrasound scanning in the diagnosis of space occupying lesions of the upper abdomen. Br J Radiol 44: 24–36, 1971.
6. Melki G: Ultrasonic patterns of tumors of the liver. JCU 1: 306–314, 1974.
7. Scheible W, Gosink BB, Leopold GG: Gray scale echographic patterns of hepatic metastatic disease. AJR 129: 983–987, 1977.
8. Green B, Bree RL, Goldstein M, Stanley C: Gray scale ultrasound evaluation of hepatic neoplasms: patterns and correlations. Radiology 124: 203–208, 1977.
9. Nicholas D: Ultrasonic diffraction analysis in the investigation of liver disease. Br J Radiol 52: 949–961, 1979.
10. Fredele MP, Filly RA, Moss AA: Cystic hepatic neoplasms: complementary roles of CT an sonography. AJR 136: 345–348, 1981.
11. Sullivan DC, Taylor LJW, Gottschald A: The use of ultrasound to enhance the diagnostic utility of equivocal liver scintigraphy. Radiology 128: 727–732, 1978.
12. Boultbee JE: Grey scale ultrasound appearances in hepatocellular carcinoma. Clin Radiol 30: 547–552, 1979.
13. Garrett WJ, Kossoff G, Uren RF, et al: Gray scale ultrasonic investigation of focal defects on 99mTc sulphur colloid liver scanning. Radiology 119: 425–428, 1976.
14. Cooperberg PL, David KB, Sauerbrei EE: Abdominal and peripheral applications of real-time ultrasound. Radiol Clin North Am 18: 59–77, 1980.
15. Kamin PD, Bernardino ME, Green B: Ultrasound manifestations of hepatocellular carcinoma. Radiology 131: 459–461, 1979.
16. Eggel H: Über das primäre Carcinom der Leber. Beitr Path Anat u z Allg Path 30: 506–604, 1901.
17. Dubbins PA, Oriordan D, Melia WM: Ultrasound in hepatoma. can specific diagnosis be made? Br J Radiol 54: 307–311, 1981.
18. Behan M, Kazan E: The echographic characteristics of fatty tissues and tumors. Radiology 129: 143–151, 1978.
19. Gosink BB, Lemon SK, Scheible W, et al: Accuracy of ultrasonography in diagnosis of hepatocellular disease. AJR 133: 19–23, 1979.
20. Harbin WP, Robert NJ, Ferrucci JT: Diagnosis of cirrhosis based on regional changes in hepatic morphology. Radiology 135: 273–283, 1980.
21. Schabe SI, Rittenberg GM, Javid LH, et al: The "bull's-eye" falciform ligament: a sonographic finding of portal hypertension. Radiology 136: 157–159, 1980.
22. Watson RC, Baltaxe HA: The angiographic appearance of primary and secondary tumors of the liver. Radiology 101: 539–548, 1971.
23. Gates GF: Atlas of Abdominal Ultrasonography in Children. New York, Churchill Livingstone, 1978.

24. Sonnenberg EV, Ferrucci JT: Bile duct obstruction in hepatocellular carcinoma (hepatoma)—clinical and cholangiographic characteristics. Report of 6 cases and review of the literature. Radiology 130: 7–13, 1979.

25. Jurio III S, Kim HS: Extrahepatic biliary obstruction by hepatocellular carcinoma. Am J Gastroenterol 74: 176–178, 1980.

26. Dubbins P, Nunnerley HB: Intratumor gas: an ultrasound sign of tumor necrosis. Clin Radiol 31: 711–715, 1980.

27. Katragadda CS, Goldstein HM, Green B: Gray scale ultrasonography of calcified liver metastasis. AJR 129: 591–593, 1977.

28. Feldman M: Hemangioma of the liver. Am J Clin Pathol 29: 160–162, 1958.

29. Winer SN, Parulekar SG: Scintigraphy and ultrasonography of hepatic hemangioma. Radiology 132: 149–153, 1979.

30. Itai Y, Furui S, Araki T, et al: Computed tomography of cavernous hemangioma of the liver. Radiology 137: 149–155, 1980.

31. Sandler MA, Peyrecelli RD, Marks DS, et al: Ultrasonic features and radionuclide correlation in liver cell adenoma and focal nodular hyperplasia. Radiology 135: 393–397, 1980.

32. Grossman H, Ram PC, Coleman RA, et al: Hepatic ultrasonography in type 1 glycogen storage disease (von Gierke disease). Radiology 141: 753–756, 1981.

33. Tesluk H, Lawrie J: Hepatocellular adenoma: Its transformation to carcinoma in a user of oral contraceptives. Arch Pathol Lab Med 105: 296–299, 1981.

34. Newlin N, Silver TM, Stuck KJ, et al: Ultrasonic features of pyogenic liver abscesses. Radiology 139: 155–159, 1981.

35. Ralls PW, Meyers HI, Lapin SA, et al: Gray-scale ultrasonography of hepatic amoebic abscesses. Radiology 132: 125–129, 1979.

36. Snow JH, Doldstein HM, Wallace S: Comparison of scintigraphy, sonography, and computed tomography in the evaluation of hepatic neoplasms. AJR 132: 915–918, 1979.

37. Miller JH: The ultrasonographic appearance of cystic hepatoblastoma. Radiology 138: 141–143, 1981.

38. Rosenbaum DM, Mindell HJ: Ultrasonographic findings in mesenchymal hamartoma of the liver. Radiology 138: 425–427, 1981.

39. Prando A, Goldstein HM, Bernardino ME, et al: Ultrasonic pseudo-lesions of the liver. Radiology 130: 403–407, 1979.

40. Broderick TW, Gosink B, Menuck L, et al: Echographic and radionuclide detection of hepatoma. Radiology 135: 149–151, 1980.

41. Hillman BJ, Smith EH, Gammelgaard J, et al: Ultrasonographic-pathologic correlation of malignant hepatic masses. Gastrointest Radiol 4: 361–365, 1979.

42. Calder JF: Ultrasound in hepatoma. Br J Radiol 54: 819, 1981.

43. Braag DG: Tumor imaging in diagnostic radiology. Cancer 47: 1159–1163, 1981.

44. McArdle CR: Ultrasonic diagnosis of liver metastases. JCU 4: 265–268, 1976.

9

ULTRASONIC DIFFERENTIAL DIAGNOSIS OF LIVER METASTASES

David O. Cosgrove

Liver metastases are of great significance in indicating the spread of a remote cancer, but their detection presents one of the most difficult problems faced by an abdominal imaging department. Improved techniques, however, have increased the accuracy of detection and characterization of liver lesions, and ultrasonography is at the forefront of these techniques.

A measure of the significance of liver metastases is their incidence at the time of discovery of the primary tumor. The incidence ranges from 1% for carcinoma of the breast to as much as 34% for melanoma. Carcinoma of the bronchus and the non-Hodgkin's lymphomas have a presentation incidence of liver metastases of about 15%. At autopsy, the great majority of tumor types are shown to be accompanied by liver metastases (1).

Liver metastases characteristically are multiple, and a single patient often shows a spectrum of sizes, suggesting sequential seeding over a period of time rather than batch seeding, which size uniformity would indicate. To some extent, the ultrasound appearances relate to the size of the metastasis, and this spread of sizes underlies the variety of echo patterns that are sometimes encountered within an involved liver.

GENERAL ULTRASONOGRAPHIC FEATURES OF LIVER METASTASES

The great majority of metastases to the liver form as focal deposits, displacing liver tissue. Detection by ultrasonography, as by other imaging techniques, depends on demonstration of the effects of these expanding lesions or on the detection of structure changes as liver tissue is replaced by tumor (Table 1).

Mass Effects

Hepatomegaly is the most direct effect of expanding lesions in the liver, but marked involvement without liver enlargement occasionally occurs. Liver size

123

TABLE 1. Features of Liver Metastases

Hepatomegaly	
Contour changes	Surface convexity/lobulation
Anatomical distortion	Displaced vessels
	lobar biliary obstruction
Focal texture changes	Reduction in echoes
	increase in echoes
	target lesions
	cystic and necrotic foci
	calcific foci

is rather difficult to assess ultrasonographically. Volume measurements of the liver, though feasible, are tedious and have not gained acceptance for routine studies. A linear dimension that can be useful is the superoinferior depth of the liver measured in the midhepatic line (2). This line midway between the midspine and the lateral margin of the liver (Figure 1) should measure less than 13 cm. A measurement greater than 15.5 cm is considered abnormal in 80% of cases. By this measurement, some 25% of cases fall into the equivocal range, as might be expected from the wide normal variation of liver shape.

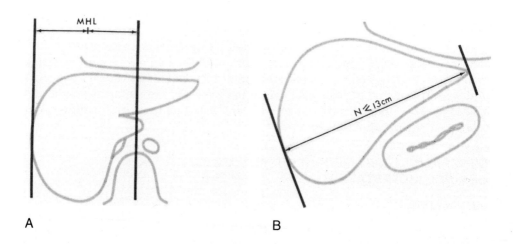

A   B

Figure 1. Measurement of liver size. The midhepatic line lies half the distance between the midspine and the lateralmost extent of the right lobe of the liver; it can be located on a transverse scan (A). The longitudinal extent of the liver in the midhepatic line is less than 13 cm in 93% of normal persons and over 15.5 cm in 75% of patients with hepatomegaly (B). Intermediate measurements are considered equivocal. MHL, midhepatic line.

The liver surface normally is smooth, convex on the anterior and diaphragmatic surfaces and gently concave on the visceral (inferoanterior) surface. In the presence of metastases there may be an alteration in these outlines, with increasing convexity. In addition, it is sometimes possible to discern sharper local convexities or lobulations overlying individual tumor masses. Both of these changes are nonspecific, being found in several nonmalignant conditions (cf. section on differential diagnosis below). Lobulations on the superior and lateral surfaces due to prominent diaphragmatic leaflets are normal and must not be mistaken for tumor masses (3) (Figure 2).

Space-occupying lesions, as well as distorting the liver outline, may distort the liver's internal anatomy. Since the vascular arrangement in the normal liver varies moderately, distortion must be marked before it can be recognized with confidence, but a displaced portal or hepatic vein sometimes is a clue that a mass lesion is present (Figure 3). Obstruction of the biliary tree, a more common sign, can be detected by the visualization of the dilated biliary vessel running alongside the portal vein branch it accompanies, so that two vessels can be seen where normally only one is present. Intrahepatic mass lesions may produce bile duct dilatation of segmental distribution without jaundice; tumor in the nodes at the porta hepatis may obstruct the common hepatic duct when generalized dilatation with jaundice develops. (The other main cause of jaundice is overall liver decompensation due to massive replacement of the liver by tumor. Rarely, jaundice due to obstruction at the cannilicular level occurs, especially in Hodgkin's disease.)

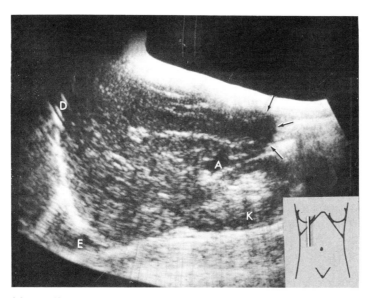

Figure 2.   Mass effect—surface distortion. The normally sharp inferior margin of the liver is rounded and convex (arrows) due to the presence of an echo-poor mass metastatic from a carcinoma of the breast. There is also a trace of ascites (A) and a small pleural effusion (E). D, diaphragm; K, right kidney. (The vertical marks are 1 cm apart in this and the following figures).

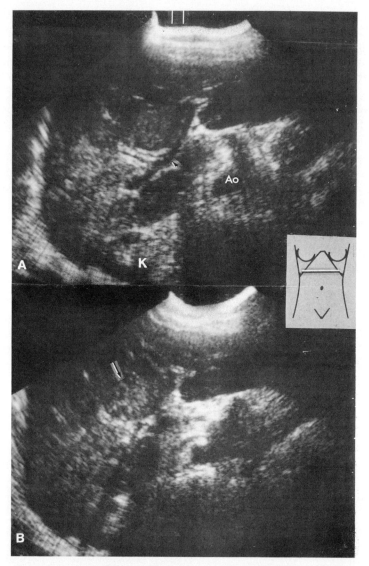

Figure 3.   Mass effect—vascular distortion. These transverse sections through a liver with multiple metastases show splaying of the portal vein (arrowhead in *A*) with posterior displacement of the right main branch due to a deposit in the quadrate lobe, which is more clearly seen in *B* (arrow). Ao, aorta; K, right kidney.

Texture Changes

Ultrasonography is sensitive to the gross physical structure of tissues. Tumors usually differ markedly from normal liver in their stiffness or elasticity and this probably causes the alterations in echo texture that are characteristic of tumors. The range of changes (Table 1) is somewhat startling and by no means fully understood, but a beginning may be made by extrapolating from basic acoustical principles. In general, since echoes are only produced by interfaces, tissues that are uniform and devoid of fibrous tissue tend to produce low-level echoes, whereas tissues with many interfaces due to fibrous or fatty tissue or to regions of hemorrhage or necrosis produce strong or plentiful echoes (4). Tumors (both primary and secondary) may be extremely homogeneous when examined under the low-power microscope, consisting of sheets of evenly spaced cells with scanty, thin-walled blood vessels. To the naked eye, the cut surface is whitish and uniform. They may also be very heterogeneous, with islands of cells surrounded by dense, reactive fibrous tissue interspersed with irregular necrotic or hemorrhagic zones that give the cut surface a complex, geographic pattern. This heterogeneous pattern corresponds to tumors that return high-level echoes (Figure 4), while tumors of the homogeneous pattern are relatively devoid of echoes (Figure 5). Smaller deposits and, especially, lymphoma nodules fall into the latter category, while the larger tumors, especially carcinomas from the gut and from the urogenital tract, more often give rise to the echo-rich type of deposit. These appearances can be useful in pointing the way to a likely primary site in the occasional patient presenting with metastases, but the chief significance of these various appearances is that they all can be due to metastases. A particularly eye-catching type of deposit is the "target lesion," which has an echo-poor peripheral band around an echo-rich center (Figure 6). Zonal necrosis or marginal sinus (venous) ectasia seems to be responsible.

The echo-poor type of deposit is the most common but the echo-rich type is seen almost as often. When there is massive replacement of liver tissue by metastases, the disrupted echo pattern is so disorganized that it is impossible to determine what is residual, viable liver and what is tumor (moth-eaten appearance, Figure 7).

Another type of deposit shows fluid features as evidenced by echo-free regions with distal enhancement due to the low attenuation of ultrasound by fluid (Figure 8). Two patterns occur. In one, the margins of the fluid are smooth and the lesion sonographically appears to be a cyst. These cystic lesions are produced by well-differentiated deposits from mucin-secreting primary sites such as the colon, the pancreas and the ovary. The second pattern corresponds to lesions that have undergone massive necrosis. Such lesions are characterized by shaggy irregular walls and the presence of echogenic debris within the fluid, which often layers out in the dependent part of the lesion. Large lesions and those under treatment are especially prone to necrose.

A rare form of metastatic involvement of the liver is seen as numerous minute (miliary) nodules scattered throughout the liver parenchyma. No focal changes are seen, but the overall liver texture becomes finer, with small closely packed echoes. Fatty change and some other diffuse infiltrations may give a similar appearance (5).

DIFFERENTIAL DIAGNOSIS OF LIVER METASTASES BY ULTRASONOGRAPHY

Liver metastases must be distinguished from normal structures that have been aptly named "pseudolesions" (6). Pseudolesions producing high-level echoes

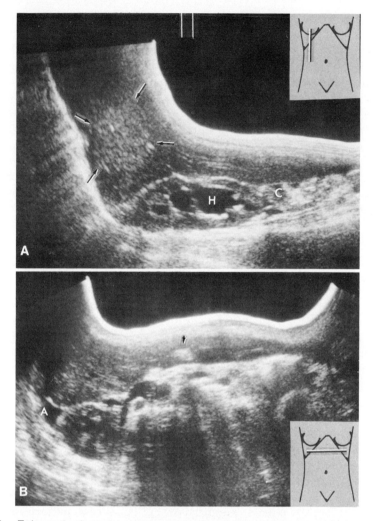

Figure 4. Echogenic deposit and the round ligament. In *A*, a large echogenic lesion (arrows) in the right lobe of the liver is shown. This tumor was a metastasis from an ovarian primary, a pelvic recurrence of which had also obstructed the right ureter, leading to gross hydronephrosis (H). In *B*, a trace of ascites (A) is shown as well as the round ligament (arrowhead), which should not be confused with a small deposit. C, ascending colon.

can simulate echogenic deposits. The most common of these is the ligamentum teres, the fibrotic, fatty remnant of the obliterated umbilical vein (Figure 4). It runs from the umbilicus in the margin of the falciform ligament, passes through the liver margin and attaches to the left portal vein. This remnant forms the boundary between the medial and lateral segments of the left lobe and may be found at or to the right of the midline. Seen in cross section on transverse views, it appears as an echogenic ovoid, whereas in longitudinal section it forms a linear echogenic streak. When it is markedly fibrotic, distal shadowing may occur. Its relationship to the portal vein and the liver margin,

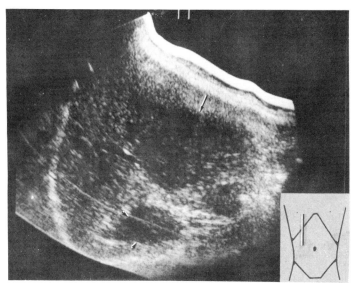

Figure 5. Echo-poor deposit. In this longitudinal section in a patient with a carcinoma of the bronchus, a large echo-poor deposit is seen (arrow); there is also a smaller lesion adjacent to it. However, the partially viewed right kidney (arrowheads) should not be confused with another deposit.

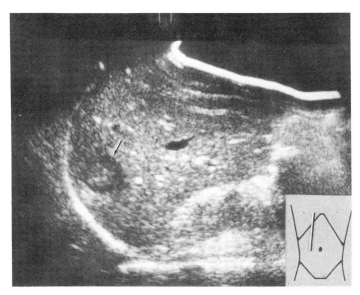

Figure 6. Target lesions. The well-defined echo-poor halo (arrow) surrounding this lesion is characteristic of a target metastasis.

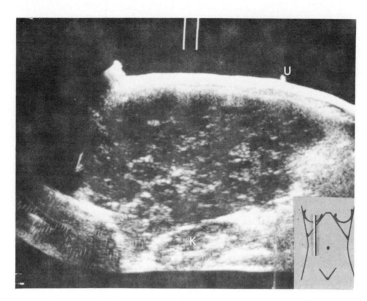

Figure 7. Extensive metastases. When the liver tissue is widely replaced by tumor tissue, the ultrasonogram takes on a disrupted or "moth-eaten" appearance, as in this example from a patient with carcinoma of the breast. K, kidney; U, level of umbilicus.

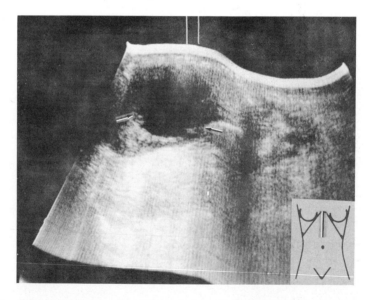

Figure 8. Necrotic metastasis. Necrosis in a tumor produces the same spectrum of ultrasonic appearances as an abscess. In this example from a patient with a carcinoma of the cervix, the distinction from a simple cyst or a secretory tumor deposit is made on the basis of the irregularities of the wall of the lesion (arrows).

both seen in longitudinal section and most easily appreciated with real-time scanning, enable the sonographer to distinguish it from a true lesion.

Several poorly reflective regions in the liver can cause confusion, the most common being simply regions of shadowing distal to the porta hepatis or the neck of the gallbladder and low-echo regions due to poor technique (loss of contact or mis-set swept gain factors). When the perirenal fat is not prominent, the cortex of the upper pole of the right kidney can produce low-level echoes that simulate a lesion in the posterior part of the right lobe of the liver. Serial sections will resolve any confusion caused by this pseudolesion, as will careful real-time scanning during deep breathing, when the greater movement of the intraperitoneal liver causes it to slide across the more fixed retroperitoneal kidney. A confusing image is sometimes produced in the superior central portion of the liver where the terminal portions of the hepatic veins produce echo-poor regions that may simulate lesions. The common portion of the left and middle hepatic veins may be surprisingly large, as may be the terminal right hepatic vein, measuring up to 2 cm in diameter. Since sonographically their walls are relatively inapparent, they may be mistaken for cystic or echo-poor structures, unless traced with serial scans.

Some normal parts of the liver may be mistaken for extrahepatic structures. The caudate lobe, a small leftward extension of the superior part of the right lobe, is separated from the posterior surface of the left lobe by a peritoneal membrane (the lesser omentum). In longitudinal section it can be mistaken for a preaortic or precaval mass, such as enlarged lymph nodes. Since the omental fat may attenuate the sound beam sufficiently to make the caudate lobe seem to have a lower level of echoes than nearby liver, this mistake is easily made (Figure 9). When the inferior vena cava lies in a deep fossa on

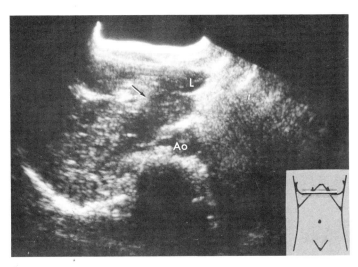

Figure 9. Caudate lobe metastasis. Because the echo levels from the caudate lobe may be lower than those from the remainder of the liver, perhaps because of attenuation due to the fissure containing the ligamentum venosum anterior to it, lesions here may be difficult to detect. In this patient with a carcinoma of the breast, however, the caudate lobe is obviously enlarged (arrow) and distorts the left lobe (L). Ao, aorta.

the posterior surface of the right lobe, the longitudinal scan through it may pick up the most medial portion of the right lobe as an apparently isolated mass of tissue in the postcaval position. In transverse section the posterior part of the left lobe sometimes seems to lie posterior to the liver and can be mistaken for stomach or another viscus. This error is made because the left portal vein, which runs transversely and may be prominent, is mistaken for the posterior surface of the liver itself. It can be avoided by examining the area in longitudinal section.

The alterations in the liver produced by metastases are by no means specific. Hepatomegaly and the increasing convexity of liver outlines can be produced by many other conditions, and focal convexities are seen in granulomata, benign tumors and, most commonly, in macronodular cirrhosis, especially in the presence of ascites. The distortion of internal structures also is nonspecific, occurring with any space-occupying lesion.

The altered echo textures perhaps are more specific, especially when taken in the context of the patient's clinical condition. Echogenic foci, however, can also be produced by gas within the liver, usually in the biliary tree, and by calcified or fibrotic granulomata or traumatic scars. More troublesome are the echogenic lesions due to the capillary type of hemangioma, which appear identical to echogenic tumors. Echo-poor foci with poorly defined margins and no distal enhancement, the most common metastatic pattern, also occur in hemangiomata of the cavernous variety. The possibility that a suspected tumor is a hemangioma is problematical when fine-needle aspiration is being considered as a diagnostic measure. One is reluctant to puncture a hemangioma, even though experience has shown hemorrhagic complications to be rare in the instances in which it has been done inadvertently. Pulsed Doppler signals and digital subtraction arteriography can aid in this situation. Multiple hemangiomata may produce a replaced or moth-eaten liver pattern, as may conditions with extensive patchy liver necrosis, such as toxic hepatitis (most commonly seen in alcoholic hepatitis), severe viral hepatitis and the multiple abscesses of severe ascending cholangitis. Patients with these diseases are usually very ill and icteric, with liver tenderness, whereas patients with hemangiomatosis are quite well. Patients with multiple liver metastases are often surprisingly well, and the liver usually is not tender.

Liver abscesses evolve through a series of ultrasonic appearances that can be rather confusing. When examined very early, all that may be seen is an ill-defined echo-poor zone. Usually rather rapidly, within days, this zone develops a well-marked echo-poor perimeter, which at this stage simulates a target metastasis. Then, as necrosis and pus form, the center becomes patchily or entirely echo free, usually with some debris, and distal enhancement develops. At this stage, the fluid-filled lesion, with its shaggy cortex of edematous, inflamed tissue, exactly simulates a necrotic tumor. Finally, an abscess may resolve by absorption or shrink to a scar that may simulate an echogenic deposit. Another end result is the formation of a postinfective, sterile cyst that is indistinguishable from a simple, developmental cyst. Thus, the ultrasound distinction between an abscess and a malignancy in the liver may be very difficult when based on a single examination. However, there usually is local tenderness over an abscess that can be pinpointed by using the ultrasonic probe as a palpator. With tumors this tenderness is found much less often. More reliable is the rapid evolution of an abscess so that a rescan the following day will usually show a marked change. Fine-needle aspiration is definitive.

Hematomas also go through a series of appearances (9). A fresh hemorrhage is virtually echo free, but within hours echogenic regions appear, sometimes showing a reflective cortex representing fibrin organization. As clot retraction and fibrosis develop, fluid regions with strands of echogenic material form. Healing results either in an echogenic scar or in a posttraumatic cyst, the features and differential considerations being the same as with a healed abscess.

Both benign tumors (10) and primary carcinomas (hepatocellular carcinomas and cholangiocarcinomas) may produce all of the signs of solid metastases and usually cannot be distinguished ultrasonographically (see Chapter II-4).

The similarity between the ultrasonic appearance of abscesses and hematomas and necrotic tumors has been mentioned. The appearance of the secretory type of cystic deposit, that arising from mucin-producing primary tumors, often is identical to that of a simple cyst. Sometimes a distinction can be made because a malignant cyst may have a patchily thickened wall. A particular problem in this context is the hydatid cyst. Two major forms may be encountered. Nonreproducing cysts have smooth walls and ultrasonographically are seen as simple cysts. Hydatid cysts reproduce by internal budding to form increscences that round off to give the pathognomonic cyst-within-a-cyst pattern. Since the simple solitary cyst type is not necessarily sterile, biopsy should be avoided. Serological studies are recommended before a biopsy sample is taken from a liver cyst in a patient from a hydatid-endemic region.

This discussion of the similarity in appearance of nonmalignant and metastatic lesions may seem to paint a hopeless picture for ultrasound diagnosis. In practice, however, the sonographer's burden is eased by the clinical context and by the fact that liver metastases only rarely are solitary. Different deposits within the same liver often produce different ultrasonographic images. Since this is not true of most benign lesions, this is a helpful point of distinction. When doubt persists and if fine-needle aspiration is undesirable (11), the relentless, slow deterioration of liver metastases is characteristic.

CLINICAL ROLE OF ULTRASOUND IMAGING IN DETECTING LIVER METASTASES

Numerous reports on the accuracy of ultrasonography in the detection of liver metastases indicate an accuracy rate of about 85%, with a marked historical trend toward improvement, due no doubt to a combination of better techniques and improved ultrasound equipment (1). However, two points are repeatedly mentioned: the intrinsic difficulty of this application of ultrasound and the lack of an adequate yardstick by which to assess the accuracy of ultrasonographic diagnosis of focal liver disease. The latter problem is especially pressing for early disease, since the sampling errors of conventional liver biopsy mean that a negative is almost without significance. Even laparotomy is inadequate, since only superficial and larger deep-seated lesions can be detected.

Autopsy, of course, is relevant as a yardstick only for late disease, which is both easier to detect and less clinically important. For these reasons the reports on the accuracy of imaging in general for focal liver disease should be regarded as provisional only.

Lesions are missed by ultrasound imaging chiefly because of a combination of small size and low contrast. Where high contrast is present, as with a strongly echogenic deposit, lesions as small as 1 cm can be detected (Figure 10). Most deposits differ but little in reflectivity from the surrounding parenchyma and so must be larger to be detectable. A realistic minimum size for the usual echo-poor deposit is 2 cm, but even much larger lesions can be quite undetectable by ultrasonography, simply because their echo levels are almost identical to those of the surrounding normal liver. Since liver metastases usually are multiple and the echo properties of the individual lesions are often different, accurate patient diagnosis is easier than the detection of each and every lesion. Careful technique is required in this exacting application, both to be sure that the whole liver, including the relatively inaccessible anterior and lateral region, has been scanned and to maximize the display of lesions imaged. In this regard, strong signal compression is preferred since it enhances small differences in reflectivity. This can be achieved by the use of preprocessing and postprocessing facilities (cf. Chapter I-4).

Published reports show a low false-positive range for ultrasound diagnosis (taking a true positive as an index of any focal disease—not necessarily tumor). Computerized tomography (CT) also produces few false-positive diagnoses, whereas isotope scanning of the conventional gamma camera type is subject to false positives due to confusing anatomical variants and also provides a large number of equivocal diagnoses. The number of lesions missed by isotope

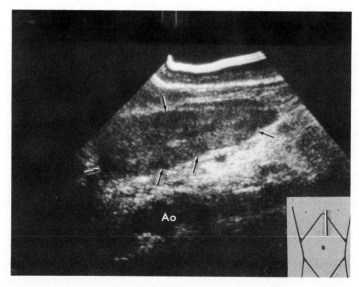

Figure 10.   Small, echo-poor metastases. Numerous lesions (arrows) can be discerned in this liver; several are associated with surface nodularity. The smallest measures approximately 1 cm.

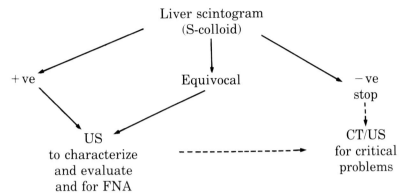

Figure 11. Investigative pathway for diagnosing focal liver lesions. US, ultrasonography; CT, computerized tomography; FNA, fine needle aspiration.

imaging is about the same as that missed by ultrasound and CT; since the isotope scan is the simplest technique, it is the preferred general screening test for focal disease in the liver. Ultrasound diagnosis should then be used for equivocal regions and to help further characterize lesions as well as to guide fine-needle aspiration. CT is reserved for critical applications or situations in which an ultrasound examination is technically impossible. An example of a critical application is the patient with a strongly suggestive clinical picture in whom the ultrasound scan is negative. The patient being screened for a partial hepatectomy for a supposed solitary metastasis in whom ultrasound is negative in the portion of liver to be left is another example. Since a negative ultrasound scan cannot be considered definitive, such a study should be supported by a CT examination with contrast medium. The flow diagram in Figure 11 is tentatively proposed as an ideal; local conditions of skill and equipment will necessarily dictate an elastic interpretation. Improvements in technology will also change the preferred sequencing. Developments offering the promise of being helpful in diagnosing focal liver disease inclue isotope CT, tumor-specific labeled-antibody scanning agents, improved ultrasound equipment, including Doppler imaging, tissue characterization and computer enhancement of ultrasound images. Conventional x-radiology may well have more to offer with the advent of digital subtraction angiography, and the development of liver contrast agents for x-ray CT may become important.

REFERENCES

1. Cosgrove DO: Liver. In Goldberg BB (ed): Ultrasound in Cancer, Clinics in Diagnostic Ultrasound, Vol 6. New York, Churchill Livingstone, 1981, pp 1–21.

2. Gosink BB, Laymaster CR: The ultrasonic determination of hepatomegaly. J Clin Ultrasound 9: 37–41, 1981.

3. Weill FS: Ultrasonography of Digestive Diseases, Chap 8, St. Louis, The CV Mosby Co, 1978.

4. Rubaltelli L, Del Maschio A, Candiani F, et al: The role of vascularisation in the

formation of echographic patterns of hepatic metastases. Br J Radiol 53: 1166–1170, 1980.

5.   Cosgrove DO, McCready VR: Diffuse metastatic disease in the liver. In White DN, Barnes RE (eds): Ultrasound in Medicine, Vol 3A. New York, Plenum Press, 1977, pp 465–466.

6.   Prando A, Goldstein HM, Bernadino ME: Ultrasonic pseudolesions in the liver. Radiology 130: 403–404, 1979.

7.   Weiner SN, Parulekar SG: Scintigraphy and ultrasound of hepatic haemangioma. Radiology 132: 149–153, 1979.

8.   Dewbury KC, Joseph AEA, Millward-Sadler GIF, et al: Ultrasound in the diagnosis of early liver abscesses. Br J Radiol 53: 1160–1166, 1980.

9.   Wicks JD, Silver TM, Bree RL: Ultrasonic features of haematomas. Am J Roentgenol 131: 977–979, 1978.

10. Atkinson GO, Kodroff M, Sones PJ, et al: Focal nodular hyperplasia of the liver in children. Radiology 137: 171–174, 1980.

11. Nosher JL, Plafker J: Fine needle aspiration of the liver with ultrasound guidance. Radiology 137: 177–180, 1980.

10

ULTRASONIC DIAGNOSIS OF GALLBLADDER CANCER

Yasuaki Takehara

EQUIPMENT

Ultrasonographic examination of the gallbladder has generally been by contact compound scanning. This technique has the advantage of providing high-quality images and a wide viewing area in one scanning process. The method unfortunately is not particularly effective for examination of organs such as the gallbladder, whose location varies among patients and is easily shifted by positional changes or respiratory movements. Effective gallbladder examination requires clear, well-defined images observed in real time with a transducer that is easy to handle. The transducer must be thin because scanning frequently must be performed through a narrow intercostal echo window (1).

Experience has shown that linear-array scanning equipment with high resolution meets these conditions. The mean detectability of gallbladders is 85% by the conventional technique and 99.5% by linear-array scanning (Table 1) (2).

PREPARATION

The most important condition for obtaining a clear image of the digestive system, including the gallbladder, is the absence of bowel gas. The fundus of the gallbladder, especially, often cannot be visualized because of gas. Therefore, the most desirable time for the examination is early, after morning fasting, when the gallbladder is not contracted. The gallbladder wall appears thickened when the gallbladder is contracted. An enema may be necessary when the patient has bowel gas and is constipated. As shown in Table 1, the detectability of the gallbladder by linear-array scanning after morning fasting is 99.5%, whereas before dinner it decreases to 92.5% (3).

137

TABLE 1.   Comparison of Echography and Oral Cholangiography for Detection of Gallbladder

	Detectability of Gallbladder	Preparation
Echography (electronic linear scanning)	99.5% (209/210) 92.5% (74/80)	Fasting in the morning Before dinner in the evening
Oral cholangiography (sodium iopodate)	94.3% (198/210)	Fasting in the morning

SCANNING METHOD AND NORMAL PATTERN

The examination usually is performed using right subcostal and right intercostal scanning. The whole gallbladder is observed by gradually changing the beam direction while the patient breaths deeply. It is necessary to rotate the transducer slightly to observe the neck and fundus of the gallbladder. The relationship between the scanning position and the displayed image is shown in Figure 1. With right intercostal scanning, the right branch of the portal vein (PV) can be observed in the inferior part of the gallbladder, as shown in Figure 1A. The right anterior inferior, the right posterior inferior and right posterior superior of the PV also are usually displayed. With right subcostal scanning, the left branch of the PV, which is located horizontally in the inferior part of the gallbladder, and the pars umbilicalis of the PV, which rises toward the abdominal wall, can be recognized, as illustrated in Figure 1B. The gallbladder is identified on the basis of these PV branches. The bilateral hepatic duct and common hepatic duct are recognized in the superior area of the branches of the portal vein (Figure 2). However, the intrahepatic bile duct is not displayed as a ductal structure unless the bile duct is dilated.

An echo from the ligamentum teres hepatis often is a cause of misdiagnosis. This echo is displayed as a high, round image at the left side of the gallbladder and at the right side of the pars umbilicalis of the PV (Figure 3). Artifacts caused by multiple reflection or a side lobe also can cause misdiagnosis. An artifact caused by multiple reflection often appears inside the gallbladder, and may be mistaken for echoes caused by pus, concentrated bile or debris (Figure 4) (4). An artifact caused by a side lobe may appear at the curved portion of the gallbladder image and around a gallstone echo and may also resemble echoes from debris (Figures 5 and 16) (5).

ECHOGRAM OF CANCER OF THE GALLBLADDER

Cancer of the gallbladder often is discovered only after symptoms of obstructive jaundice or of a mass in the right hypochondral region appear. In most cases, a radical operation cannot be performed because the lesion has not been discovered. Conventional cholangiographies, which display the biliary system by

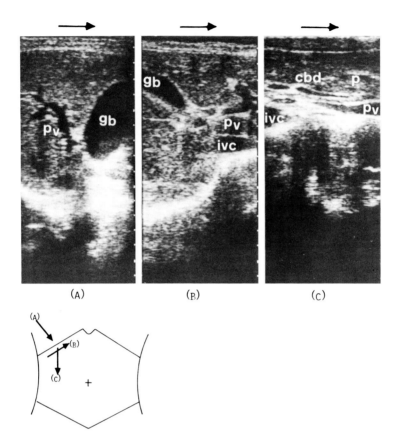

(A)   (B)   (C)

Figure 1. Relationship between the scanning position and the displayed image. Pv, portal vein; gb, gallbladder; cbd, common bile duct; P, pancreas; ivc, inferior vena cava. (A) Right intercostal scan; (B) right subcostal scan; (C) longitudinal scan.

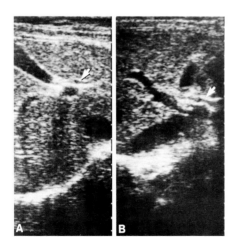

Figure 2. Echogram of bilateral hepatic duct (arrows). (A) Right subcostal scan; (B) right intercostal scan.

139

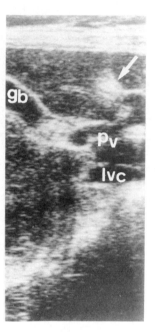

Figure 3. In the right subcostal scan, the ligamentum teres hepatis is displayed as a round, high echogenic image on the left side of the gallbladder (arrow). Ivc, Inferior vena cava; Pv, left branch of portal vein; gb, gallbladder.

utilizing a contrast medium, do not display details inside the gallbladder wall or small lesions inside the gallbladder itself. Also, when a morphological change of the gallbladder, such as obstruction of the cystic duct, occurs, contrast radiography of the interior of the gallbladder usually is not performed, and no information other than that concerning the obstruction is obtained. Because the ultrasonic examination displays a sectional view of the gallbladder without a contrast medium, it may be expected to contribute to the detection of early cancer of the gallbladder.

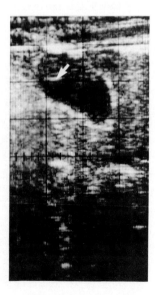

Figure 4. Artifact caused by a multiple reflection inside the gallbladder (arrow).

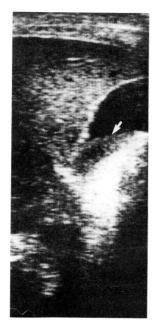

Figure 5. Artifact caused by a side lobe inside the gall-bladder (arrow).

As shown in Figure 6A-C, (6–8) the pattern of an echogram of cancer of the gallbladder from the viewpoint of tumor growth may be classified as follows (9, 10):

1) Circumscribed type (mass formation type)
A polyplike image appears inside the gallbladder (Figure 7). Most lesions of this type can be resected by operation.
2) Diffuse type (thickened wall type)
The image is of cancer infiltrating the gallbladder wall, which is thickened (Figure 8). The diffuse type is an advanced cancer that usually has directly invaded the liver.
3) Mixed type
A complicated pattern in which types 1 and 2 are mixed (Figure 9).

Most (80–90%) cancers of the gallbladder are accompanied by gallstones. Cancers with and without gallstones have different patterns. Cancers with gallstones show tumor images mixed with strong echoes caused by the gall-stones, and an acoustic shadow is seen in the inferior area (Figures 8 and 9). Cancers of the gallbladder with accompanying obstruction of the cystic duct often show weak echoes caused by concentrated bile or debris.

If gallstones or debris are present, the following characteristics must be also considered:

1) Circumscribed type (Mass formation type)
This type is displayed as an image similar to that of a deformed polyp inside the gallbladder or as a complicated, heterogeneous tumor. If it is

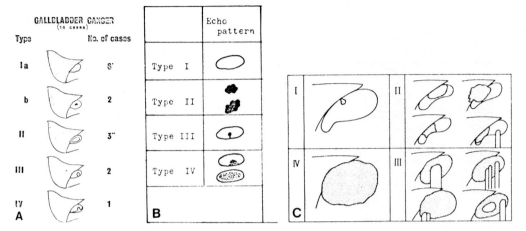

Figure 6. (A) Classification of echographic appearance of gallbladder cancer prepared by Hsu-Chong Yeh. (From Yeh HC: Ultrasonography and computed tomography of carcinoma of the gallbladder. Radiology 133: 167, 1979.) (B) Classification of echographic appearance of gallbladder cancer prepared by Watanabe E, et al. (From Watanabe E, Hongo H, Murata E, et al: Ultrasonography of carcinoma of the gallbladder. JSUM Meeting 36: 115, 1980.) (C) Classification of echographic appearance of gallbladder cancer prepared by G. Watanabe et al. (From Watanabe G, Bandai Y, Itoh T, et al: Ultrasonographic evaluation of the carcinoma of the gallbladder—4 types of gallbladder cancer of 22 cases and the analysis of the suspected cases of the gallbladder cancer. JSUM Meeting 35: 253, 1979.)

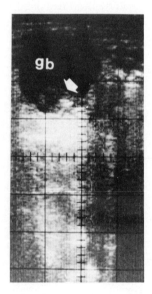

Figure 7. A gallbladder cancer echogram displaying circumscribed pattern (arrow). gb, gallbladder.

142

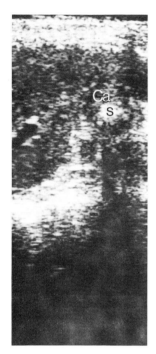

Figure 8. Echogram of cancer of the gallbladder (diffuse type). S, gallstone; Ca, cancer.

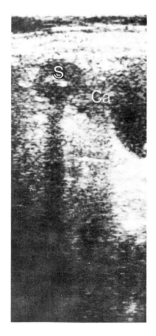

Figure 9. Echogram of cancer of the gallbladder (mixed type). S, gallstone; Ca, cancer.

143

not accompanied by a gallstone, the acoustic shadow usually does not appear. In this case, right intercostal or right subcostal scanning should be performed to prove that the tumor or polypoid image is continuous with the wall of the gallbladder. Weak echoes caused by debris around the tumor often are observed (Figure 7). These echoes show a fluid level that is affected by the scanning position (Figure 10).

2) Diffuse type (infiltrative type)
The basic findings of a cancer that does not protrude inside the gallbladder but infiltrates its wall are a thickened wall and deformation of the gallbladder. This type of cancer often is accompanied by gallstones. Unfortunately, chronic cholecystitis shows the same pattern, and differential diagnosis therefore is difficult. Cancer differs from chronic cholecystitis in that the wall of the gallbladder is not homogeneous and the inner surface (mucous membrane) is irregular (Figure 11) (11). These differences are not observed in all cases, and if the image shows a thickened wall but no signs of inflammation, aspiration cytology by echo-guided puncture must be performed (12, 13).

3) Mixed type
In this type, the cavity of the gallbladder almost disappears, and an irregular tumor image is observed (Figure 12). If the tumor is accompanied by gallstones, the pattern becomes complicated, with an acoustic shadow in the inferior area.

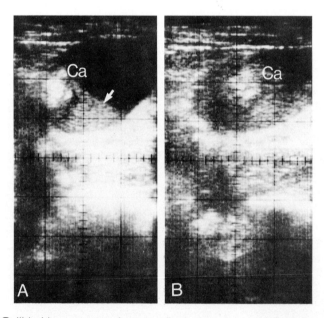

Figure 10. Gallbladder cancer echogram displaying circumscribed pattern. The echo caused by the debris forms a niveau (fluid level) (arrow). Ca, cancer. (A) Right intercostal scan; (B) right subcostal scan.

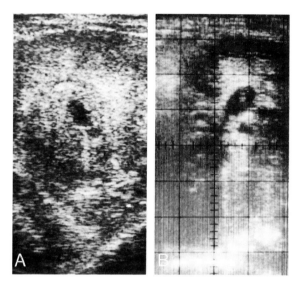

Figure 11. Comparison of the inside of the gallbladder wall in cases of gallbladder cancer (*A*) and chronic cholecystitis (*B*).

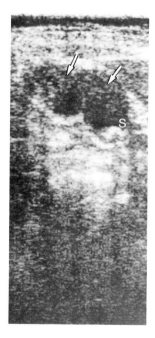

Figure 12. The gallbladder is deformed, and weak echoes (arrows) caused by cancer are seen from the fundus to the body of the gallbladder. S, gallstone.

ECHOGRAMS OF DISEASES DIFFERENTIATED FROM CANCER OF THE GALLBLADDER

Cholelithiasis

The characteristics of this disease are a strong, simple echo from the calculi and posterior acoustic shadow. It therefore is easily differentiated from cancer. Attention must be given to patients in whom many small gallstones and debris exist together. The echograms in such cases show mixed strong echoes from gallstones and weak echoes from debris (Figure 13) (14). Careful observation will show that the strong echoes are clearly separated, allowing the differentiation.

The acoustic shadow of cholelithiasis varies according to the nature and size of the gallstones. If the calculus is a combination stone or mixed stone (cholesterol-bilirubin-calcium stone), a clear acoustic shadow is present. If it is a pure pigment stone, the acoustic shadow is not as clear. In these cases caution is necessary, because the gallstone echo may be complicated and occasionally may resemble a tumor (Figure 14). The grade of acoustic shadow is related to the size of the gallstone and the width of the ultrasonic beam. With current equipment, the acoustic shadow becomes evident when the diameter of the stones exceeds 2 mm (Figure 15).

In the diagnosis of gallstones, it is important to differentiate the debris from the artifact echoes caused by side lobes, which often appear around the gallstone. The artifact is displayed symmetrically around the stone, and in this way differs from the echoes due to debris (Figure 16).

Cholecystitis

The gallbladder usually is swollen in cases of acute (Figure 17) and chronic cholecystitis (Figure 18). A thickened wall or even sometimes a double-layered

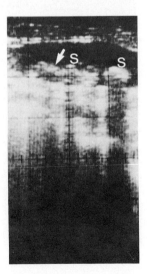

Figure 13.   Echogram of cholecystolithiasis with complicated echoes caused by debris (arrow). S, gallstone.

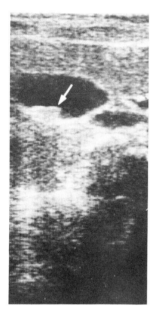

Figure 14. A pure pigment stone (arrow) is not usually accompanied by an acoustic shadow and can easily be misdiagnosed as a tumor because its echoes are displayed in a complicated pattern.

wall is seen. Weak internal echoes due to pus, concentrated bile or debris are often visible (15). These internal echoes present a fluid level that alters with the scanning position (Figure 10). In acute cholecystitis, the surrounding tissues and the wall of the gallbladder become edematous and the boundary echo of the gallbladder wall is not clear (Figure 17) (16). In acute and chronic cholecystitis, the thickened gallbladder wall is homogeneous, and the inner surface is regular, allowing it to be distinguished from diffuse cancer. When the image of a thickened gallbladder wall shows a double-layered structure, the possibility of cancer is slight. In cholecystitis, the gallbladder often is swollen,

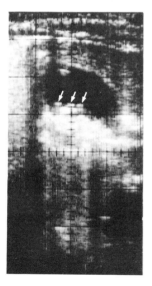

Figure 15. Small gallstones (arrows), approximately 2 mm in diameter, are not usually accompanied by an acoustic shadow.

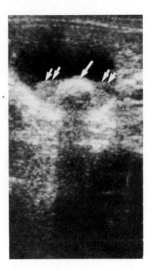

Figure 16. Artifact (small arrows) caused by a side lobe around the gallstone echo (arrow).

and sometimes the whole gallbladder cannot be displayed on the limited field of view of the array. It then is necessary to examine the gallbladder by moving the transducer so that an accompanying stone or circumscribed mass is not overlooked. Also, if the gallbladder is swollen because the gallstone is incarcerated at the neck of the gallbladder or because the tumor is in the neck of the gallbladder, dilatation of the intrahepatic bile duct (Mirrizi syndrome) (17) is often detected by pressing the common hepatic duct or common bile duct (Figure 18) (18).

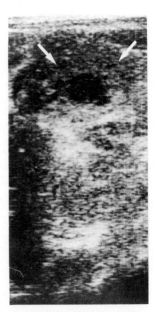

Figure 17. In cases of acute cholecystitis, the gallbladder wall is remarkably swollen (arrows) and its boundaries are not clear.

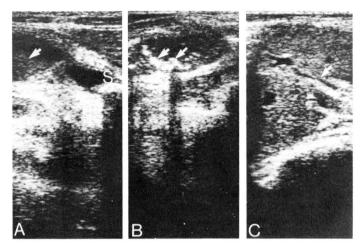

Figure 18. Echograms of chronic cholecystitis. (*A*) Thickness of the gallbladder wall and weak echoes (arrow) caused by debris can be seen. S, gallstone. (*B*) Many small stone echoes (arrows) in the fundus of the gallbladder. (*C*) Dilation of the intrahepatic bile duct (arrow).

Polypoid Lesions of the Gallbladder

The characteristics for this disease are as follows (19, 20):

1. An echo caused by polypoid lesions appears inside the gallbladder and is contiguous with the gallbladder wall. This can be proved by noting that the echo does not shift by positional changes or in response to external stimulus. A cholesterol polyp (Figure 19) has a greater tendency to move than an adenomatous or inflammatory polyp.

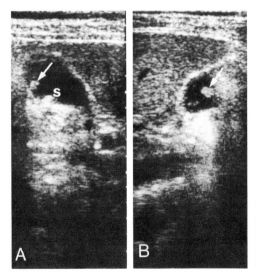

Figure 19. Echogram of a cholesterol polyp (arrow). The polyp is contiguous with the gallbladder wall. (*A*) Right subcostal scan. (*B*) Right intercostal scan. S, gallstone.

2. Even if a polypoid lesion has a diameter as large as 5 mm, no acoustic shadow is present. Previously, it was thought that there are only a few individuals with this disease in Japan. However, about 1.0% of those who have undergone echographic gallbladder survey have been found to have this disease (5.0% of them have gallstones). It is not easy to differentiate polypoid lesions from cancer. In a polypoid lesion, the tumor image that protrudes inside the gallbladder is small and homogeneous and its boundaries are regular, whereas a cancer image is heterogeneous and its boundaries are irregular. If a polypoid lesion is greater than 5 mm in diameter and the surface is slightly irregular, it should be positively resected; in other cases, follow-up echographic examinations should be conducted monthly or bimonthly. If any change is noticed, resection should be performed.

RESULTS OF A SURVEY EXAMINATION

In the past, oral cholangiography has been used for gallbladder screening. Recent results suggest that ultrasonic examinations are superior for this application since:

1) It is not necessary to use a contrast medium, and side effects can be avoided.
2) Echography is more effective in detecting the gallbladder (3).
3) Echography provides better capability for detecting small lesions such as stones and polypoid lesions (Table 2) and early cancer of the gallbladder can be detected.

**TABLE 2. Comparison of Echography and Oral Cholangiography Results*

	Oral Cholangiography	Echography by Electronic Linear Scanning	Cases
Cholecystolithiasis	●	●	3
	○	●	4
	●	○	0
Polypoid lesion of gallbladder	●	●	0
	○	●	3
	●	○	0
Other abnormal findings	●	●	0
	○	●	14†
	●	○	1
			25

* Total cases: 178
Cases diagnosed as normal by both examinations: 153
Cases in which an abnormal finding was recognized by one examination: 25

●, detected
○, not detected
†, artifact

TABLE 3.   Examination of Dry Dock Workers, November 20, 1979—July 31, 1981 (4,542 Cases)

Examination	Number of Cases	Percent of Cases
Biliary Tract		
Normal gallbladder	4109	90.5
Stone of gallbladder	236	5.2
Polypoid lesion or small stone of gallbladder	7	0.2
Polypoid lesion of gallbladder	47	1.0
Choledochal cyst	2	
Stone of extrahepatic bile duct	1	
Dilation of intrahepatic bile duct	2	
Abnormal gallbladder (re-exam)	92	2.0
Abnormal echoes	36	0.8
Wall thickness	9	0.2
Deformity	25	0.6
Judgment impossible because of gas	22	0.5
Postcholecystectomy	46	1.0
Liver		
Normal liver	4194	92.3
Fatty liver	70	1.5
Liver cyst (solitary)	85	1.9
Polycystic liver	5	0.1
Intrahepatic stone	5	0.1
Liver tumor	16	0.4
Abnormal liver (re-exam)	167	3.7
Heterogeneous intrahepatic echoes	121	2.7
Deformity	34	0.7
Judgment impossible because of gas	12	0.3
Details		
Liver cancer	3	
Hemangioma	4	
Liver cirrhosis	7	
Follow-up	2	

4)   Echography at the same time permits observation of the liver and kidneys (Table 3).

Table 1 shows a comparison of oral cholangiography and echography in detection of the gallbladder in a study in which workers in a dry dock were the subjects. The time required for echography was on the average 5 minutes per subject, including the time for preparing for examination, such as undressing and dressing. As shown in Table 2, it was found that echography was more effective for detecting gallbladder stones and polypoid lesions. Unfortunately, many false-positive errors due to artifacts echoes were made. To eliminate these false positives, it was found necessary to adopt a double-check system, in which the diagnosis was performed with real-time and static images.

Table 3 indicates the results of ultrasonic examinations of the liver and biliary tract made from November 1979–July 1981. According to a monthly analysis, the detectability of cholelithiasis, polypoid lesions and liver cysts all were constant at 5.0%, 1.0% and 2.0%, respectively. It was suspected that 16 of those examined had liver tumors. Among these were two cases of hepatoma (one case was early cancer), one of metastatic liver cancer and four hemangiomas. The remaining cases were cirrhosis of the liver. Because of the low incidence of the disease, cancer of the gallbladder was not encountered in this group.

REFERENCES

1. Takehara Y: Clinical application of real-time imaging in digestive system. In Wagai T, Omoto, R (eds.): Ultrasound in Medicine and Biology. Amsterdam, Excerpta Medica, 1980, p 168.

2. Vassilios R, Lawrence M, Karen R, et al: Comparison of real-time and gray-scale static ultrasonic cholecystography. Radiology 140: 153, 1981.

3. Takehara Y: Clinical evaluation of electronic linear scan. Jpn J Med Ultrasonics 5: 47, 1978.

4. Itoh K, Ozawa M, Oikawa T, et al: Ultrasonic diagnosis of the gallbladder carcinoma. JSUM Meeting 37: 373, 1980.

5. Takeuchi H, Takehara Y: Ultrasonic Diagnosis of Malignant Tumor. Tokyo Techno Inc, 1980.

6. Yek HC: Ultrasonography and computed tomography of carcinoma of the gallbladder. Radiology 133: 167, 1979.

7. Watanabe E, Hongo H, Murata E, et al: Ultrasonography of carcinoma of the gallbladder. JSUM Meeting 36: 115, 1980.

8. Watanabe G, Bandai Y, Itoh T, et al: Ultrasonographic evaluation of the carcinoma of the gallbladder—4 types of gallbladder cancer of 22 cases and the analysis of the suspected cases of the gallbladder cancer. JSUM Meeting 35: 253, 1979.

9. Yokomizo S, Yano M, Nakayama T, et al: Ultrasonography of the carcinoma of the gallbladder. JSUM Meeting 37: 377, 1980.

10. Watanabe E, Inayoshi A, Kanemitsu K, et al: Echo patterns of gallbladder carcinoma. JSUM Meeting 37: 375, 1980.

11. Ohashi K, Yamashita S, Yamamoto S, et al: Ultrasonogram of the gallbladder carcinoma. JSUM Meeting 38: 409, 1981.

12. Watanabe Y, Ryu M, Kikuchi T, et al: Ultrasonic diagnosis of gallbladder diseases—Study of polypoid lesion. JSUM Meeting 39: 289, 1981.

13. Awatsu R, Inoue S, Ishida H: False positive and negative cases of gallbladder carcinoma on US study. Proceedings of the Meeting of the Japan Society of Ultrasonics in Medicine (JSUM Meeting) 39: 291, 1981.

14. Kobayashi M, Takagi T, Nishihara E, et al: Diagnostic significance of ultrasound examination of the gallbladder cancer. JSUM Meeting 38: 411, 1981.

15. Lim I, Ogasawara T, Taima T, et al: Abnormal echoes in gallbladder with cholecystitis observed by S-US. JSUM Meeting 39: 287, 1981.

16. Murata Y, Abe H, Yokomichi H, et al: Ultrasonic evaluation of gallbladder wall in cholecystitis—a comparison with histopathological findings. JSUM Meeting 39: 283, 1981.

17. Dewbury KC: The features of the Mirizzi syndrome on ultrasound examination. Br J Radiol 52: 990, 1979.

18. Conrad MR, Landay MJ, Janes JO: Sonographic "parallel channel" sign of biliary tree enlargement in mild to moderate obstructive jaundice. Am J Roentgenol 130: 279, 1978.

19. Carter SJ, Rutledge J, Hirsch JH, et al: Papillary adenoma of the gallbladder. Ultrasonic demonstration. J Clin Ultrasound 6: 433, 1978.

20. Ruhe AH, Zachman JP, Mulder BD, et al: Cholesterol polyps of the gallbladder. Ultrasound demonstration. J Clin Ultrasound 7: 386, 1979.

11

ULTRASONOGRAPHY OF PANCREATIC TUMORS

George R. Leopold

Carcinoma of the pancreas has long been one of the most dreaded of the malignant neoplasms. Since the disorder often is in an advanced state when discovered, surgical cure is rare. Chemotherapy and radiation therapy usually are only palliative. To make matters worse, the incidence of this disorder has been steadily increasing over the last decade, although some believe that this is due, in part, to improved methods of diagnosis. To increase survival, it is apparent that earlier detection is much to be desired. It may well be that this detection will not be by means of an imaging method but rather by identification of subtle alterations of the body's immunochemical regulatory mechanism (1). It is clear, however, that present imaging methods, including ultrasonography, have great utility in properly staging this disorder (2). Long considered to be the "hidden organ" because of its high retroperitoneal location, the pancreas is now easily imaged by both ultrasonography and computed tomography (CT) (3). Since metastases to regional lymph nodes and the liver as well as secondary effects on the biliary tree are detectable by both methods, they are of great benefit in planning the patient's therapy. In many situations, information gained from these procedures will prevent unnecessary surgery, obviating the expense and high morbidity that attend such procedures.

SCANNING TECHNIQUES

Today's ultrasonographer has at his disposal a wide variety of instruments with which to examine the upper abdomen. This is in distinct contrast to a decade ago when only the static B-scanner with its bistable images was available. Early reports seemed to indicate that the normal pancreas and solid pancreatic tumors were only rarely visualized, while fluid-containing disease processes (pancreatitis, pseudocyst) could be detected with greater frequency. Modern instruments of both the static and real-time variety permit detailed examination of the normal pancreatic parenchyma in the great majority of cases. This is, in large measure, due to the development of sophisticated pro-

154

cessing schemes that allow presentation of returning echo information in gradations of intensity (gray-scale recording). Although at first only static scanners possessed adequate gray-scale capability, it is now apparent that many real-time instruments have achieved good image quality. Whether one uses a static or real-time scanner is not nearly as important as a detailed knowledge of the local anatomy and an understanding of the interaction between ultrasound and soft tissue. The merits and disadvantages of both types of instrument will be briefly discussed.

Static scanners have as their major benefit presentation of the image information in a relatively complete anatomic cross section. This facilitates recognition by surgeons or other individuals who were not actually present at the time of the examination. Acceptance of these studies remains somewhat higher than real-time studies, with their more limited field of view. It should be mentioned, however, that static scans achieve this completeness by compounding transducer movement, which often obscures the important information being sought. When maximum anatomic detail is desired, small sector scans are made over the area of the pancreas resulting in the same limited field of view that is obtained in real-time imaging. A complete examination of the pancreatic area might include 30 or so images—some compound and some single-sector passes. If these images are obtained by a technologist working independent of the physician performing the interpretation, the latter should be made aware that many more images were made by the former but discarded as "nondiagnostic," thus avoiding the possibility of overlooking significant information.

Real-time scanners, produce not 30–60 but literally thousands of images during the course of the examination. In addition, real-time scanning requires far less skill to produce diagnostic images than does static scanning. As mentioned above, real-time instruments have until recently suffered from lack of gray scale in captured individual frames, but this disadvantage has now been virtually eliminated. Since field of view is restricted in real-time scanning, it is desirable to have the interpretation rendered by the individual actually performing the examination. To some this will constitute a distinct disadvantage.

Real-time equipment comes in a variety of formats. Since in the examination of the pancreas access is often a problem, it is apparent that sector scanners (of both the mechanical and phased-array types) are to be preferred to linear-array scanners. Even though linear arrays are frequently too bulky to fit in the epigastrium or intercostal spaces, they can sometimes be used successfully by oblique angling beneath the ribs.

A further consideration in choice of real-time equipment is adaptability to ultrasound-guided biopsy techniques (4, 5). In general, one would like to have a detachable, disposable biopsy unit which could quickly be fitted to the transducer so that needle passage could be monitored during insertion. An alternative method, chosen by some manufacturers is to put a hole through the transducer itself. This method requires resterilization of the probe between each application. The long-term effects of cold (gas) sterilization on such sensitive electronics is not known.

PERFORMANCE OF THE EXAMINATION

The only preparation advocated for pancreatic scanning is to require the patient to fast for at least 8 hours before the examination. This allows the gallbladder to dilate to its maximum size, facilitating examination of the biliary tree. It is hoped that this will also allow the stomach to empty of air and improve visualization of the body and tail of the pancreas. Various regimens have been suggested to eliminate the interfering effects of gas-filled loops of bowel, but none of these seems to be greatly effective. Indeed, CT has shown that in many patients in whom adequate ultrasonography is not possible, it is retroperitoneal and mesenteric fat that is responsible, rather than intestinal gas (6). Such patients are excellent candidates for study by CT, which depends upon this fat to outline the retroperitoneal organs.

Some authors advocate filling the stomach with liquid to improve visualization of the various segments of the pancreas (7, 8). A variety of patient positions may then be employed to demonstrate the specific segments. With the patient supine, ingested fluid pools in the dependent fundus of the stomach (9). This maneuver facilitates inspection of the tail of the gland (Figure 1). Further filling distends the more anteriorly located gastric antrum, highlighting the body of the pancreas (Figure 2). The pancreatic head is best examined by filling the duodenal loop. This is easily achieved by placing the patient in a partial right lateral decubitus position. Scans with the patient in this position are often supplemented by erect or partially erect scans, which displace gastric air into the superior portion of the fundus (10). These positions also have the advantage of bringing the left lobe of the liver down over the pancreatic bed to serve as an additional transonic window to the area being evaluated. Although some authors place the patient in the prone position to study the region of the pancreatic tail (11), this is a relatively low-yield procedure. In addition to possible confusion with stomach and colon, the image is often degraded by the severe attenuation of the large back muscles.

The nature of the fluid used to distend the stomach is also the subject of

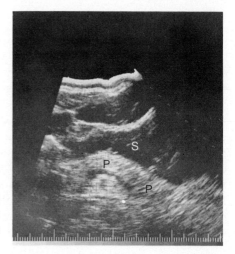

Figure 1.   Transverse scan of the upper abdomen after the stomach (S) has been filled with water. The fluid-filled stomach helps in visualizing the body and tail of the pancreas (P).

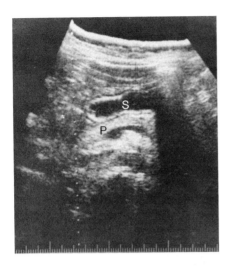

Figure 2. Transverse scan with patient rotated to the right. Filling of the gastric antrum (S) produces better visualization of the body and head of the pancreas (P).

considerable discussion. Many use ordinary tap water, while others insist that the stomach be degassed (allowed to stand for several hours) to eliminate small air bubbles. Some think that water is not a satisfactory medium, since the acoustic enhancement produced distal to it may obscure important detail in the pancreatic bed. Usually, this effect may be counteracted by reducing the overall system gain. These authors recommend a variety of fluids, including dilute solutions of methylcellulose and fruit juices (preferably containing particulate matter ["bits"] to produce some attenuation). Although fluid ingestion undoubtedly saves some ultrasonographic examinations of the pancreas and is definitely worth trying, it is not without its drawbacks. For one thing, the amount of fluid necessary is large (usually on the order of a liter) and the patient may have difficulty in accommodating it.

NORMAL ANATOMY

Pancreatic scanning is most easily performed by using the blood vessels of this area as guideposts (12). The pancreatic head is best seen on sagittal scans in the plane of the inferior vena cava. Novices are often surprised by the vertical extent of the pancreatic head. Portions of the distal aspect of the common bile duct are also frequently visualized in this plane. Once the location of the pancreatic head has been noted, transverse scans at this level are made to complete the evaluation. In many patients the pointed uncinate process of the head may be seen projecting medially behind the superior mesenteric vein. On scans of exceptionally high quality, the common bile duct may be seen within the posterior aspect of the pancreatic head. Although these orientations generally apply, anatomic variation is common, as with other abdominal viscera. For example, the pancreas lies entirely to the left of the midline in up to 5% of patients. The size of the normal pancreatic head has been discussed by many authors (13). Unfortunately, no uniform scheme has been devised for making these measurements. Many have made the mistake of making a direct anterior-

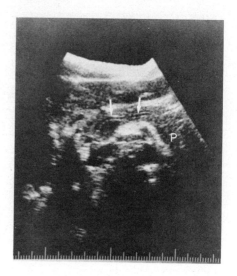

Figure 3. Transverse scan showing excellent visualization of the pancreas (P) and duct of Wirsung (arrows) in this normal subject.

posterior measurement in the region of the junction between the head and body of the gland. Since the pancreas is a curved structure, it is not surprising that spurious data have been produced. If care is taken to measure the head perpendicular to its posterior border, most authors would agree that diameters greater than 3 cm should be regarded as abnormal. As with most such measurements, the eye of the experienced observer is probably more reliable than individual measurements. Since the body of the pancreas tends to be oriented in a more horizontal plane, the best images result from scans conducted in a transverse plane. The most useful vascular marker is the splenic vein, which is closely applied to the dorsal aspect of the gland. Although it usually courses along the superior aspect of the dorsal surface, considerable variation again is common. Transverse scans just caudal to this level will show the pancreas stretched across the superior mesenteric vessels. If single-sector pass scans are employed to produce maximum resolution, the main pancreatic duct (Wirsung) is often visualized in the center of the gland. Most frequently, this will appear as an echo-dense line, representing the two walls and collapsed lumen of the duct. Sometimes, normal patients will exhibit a small amount of fluid within the lumen (Figure 3). It is stated that external diameters of the pancreatic duct in excess of 2 mm should be regarded as abnormal. Most authors have noted that the pancreatic duct is much more commonly seen in the body of the gland than in the head. This is most likely due to its favorable orientation (perpendicular) to the examining beam in this segment.

The body of the pancreas often appears to be significantly smaller in diameter than the pancreatic head and seldom exceeds 2 cm.

The pancreatic tail usually is best seen in transverse scans through a fluid-filled stomach. Vascular structures are less helpful in localization. The tail frequently is somewhat larger than the body but is also subject to variation.

When discussing the frequency of pancreatic visualization by ultrasonography, it is important to make clear which segment is being considered (14). When scanning techniques are optimal, the pancreatic head and body can be imaged in 80–85% of patients, but the pancreatic tail is visualized in no more than 30–35%. Fortunately, for ultrasonographers, pathology of the pancreatic tail is far less common than that of other segments of the gland.

Many investigators initially were puzzled by the fact that in some patients the peripancreatic vasculature could be well visualized (indicating successful penetration of the sound beam to that depth) but that the edges of the pancreas itself were not visualized. This paradox is particularly common in older patients. Recent anatomic material and CT have provided the explanation for this phenomenon. Such studies show that pancreatic fat lobules are common in the elderly, resulting in a "marbled" appearance of the gland (15, 16). This fat closely resembles the retroperitoneal fat and probably accounts for ultrasound's failure to define the margins of the gland. Although one would expect these findings in chronic atrophic pancreatitis, the same appearance is noted in many individuals with no evidence of pancreatic dysfunction.

TUMORS

Since symptoms appear relatively late in the course of pancreatic carcinoma, it is unfortunately true that many lesions are large and inoperable by the time they are discovered by sonography. The same statement applies to diagnosis by CT.

Most cancers appear as solid masses that deform the external contour of the organ (17, 18). They may involve any segment of the gland, but are most common in the pancreatic head. Although some tumors tend to be hypoechoic (Figure 4) when compared with normal parenchyma, others have a very similar texture. It should be obvious then, that small tumors that do not deform the outline of the gland will be overlooked by ultrasonography. A report of "normal pancreas" on an ultrasound study cannot be used to exclude this disorder. If

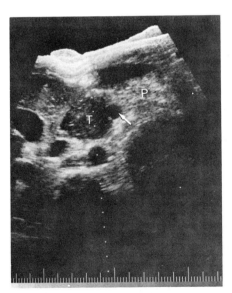

Figure 4.   Transverse scan. The head of the pancreas (P) is replaced by a tumor (T) that is relatively hypoechoic when compared with the remainder of the gland. The arrow points to the superior mesenteric vein.

the tumor is hypoechoic, then the technique may succeed in visualizing small intrapancreatic lesions where all other methods fail. Although there are many published papers claiming to evaluate the sensitivity of ultrasonography in carcinoma detection, all are flawed by variations in examiner skill, size of lesion and other factors (19–22). Sensitivity, then, can probably be defined only on a local basis for each institution. Given the ability to visualize the involved segment of the gland (see above) most experienced examiners should be able to detect a mass lesion in 85 to 90% of patients with pancreatic carcinoma.

In those patients who prove to be operable, the cancer most often turns out to be a small lesion producing obstruction of the common bile duct, the pancreatic duct, or both. In the first situation, jaundice (usually said to be painless, although often symptomatic) indicates the need for imaging studies. Some have speculated that there may be a subgroup among these patients in which only pancreatic duct dilatation initially is visualized (23, 24). Although we have identified several such patients (Figure 5), to date none has proved to be operable.

Given these pessimistic findings, it seems logical to question whether ultrasonography and CT do more than satisfy the curiosity of the physician. We believe that these techniques do play a diagnostic role in two important ways. First, the diagnosis can be made expeditiously by means of percutaneous aspiration biopsy if one uses the spatial information supplied by ultrasonography or CT. Use of the thin-walled 22 or 23 gauge Chiba needle for aspiration biopsy has proven to be both safe and accurate (25). This is an important step, since the appearance of a solid pancreatic mass itself is no guarantee that the lesion is malignant (Figure 6). Recognition of cancer cells by the pathologist skilled in cytologic techniques (a must for this procedure) proves that the mass in question is not a focal area of pancreatitis. Conversely, a diagnosis of pancreatitis in no way excludes carcinoma, since inflammatory areas often surround pancreatic tumors.

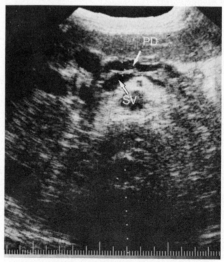

Figure 5. In this transverse scan, a dilated pancreatic duct (PD) is the only evidence of the small, unseen tumor of the pancreatic head. The splenic vein (SV) is seen in its characteristic position on the dorsal surface of the gland.

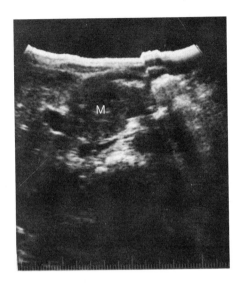

Figure 6. Transverse scan. Although this large, hypoechoic mass (M) of the pancreatic head could easily have been diagnosed as a carcinoma, it is simply a focus of chronic pancreatitis and was unchanged after 3 years.

The biopsy itself is performed with only skin anesthesia and may be done on an outpatient basis. The site, depth, and angulation of needle insertion are then ascertained from the ultrasound images. With larger lesions the procedure is easily accomplished by simply placing a mark on the skin and proceeding free hand. For somewhat smaller lesions, it may be advantageous to utilize specialized transducers through which the biopsy needle may be inserted. These are usually real-time devices that permit simultaneous visualization of the target during insertion. Although the needle itself may be difficult to see, deformation of overlying tissue planes often serves to indicate its position. To assure that adequate samples are obtained, six to eight passes with the needle are usually made.

An interesting extension of this technique has been made by Ohto et al (26), who have used real-time ultrasonography to puncture the pancreatic duct, inject radiographic contrast material and thus assist in the diagnosis of both benign and malignant disease.

Having established the diagnosis in this manner, the major advantage of ultrasonography now comes forth. A large lesion, peripancreatic adenopathy, involvement of the superior mesenteric vessels or liver metastases, all of which usually can be identified on ultrasonography, indicate inoperability. It has clearly been shown that operating on these unfortunate individuals frequently hastens their demise. Many such surgeries are performed to alleviate biliary obstruction and the severe pruritus that sometimes accompanies it, but even this can now be accomplished percutaneously (27). In this procedure, a biliary drainage catheter is passed over a guide wire that has been advanced through the obstruction into the duodenum. Numerous side holes are present, both above and below the obstruction to promote drainage.

It should be apparent that many of these patients can be diagnosed and treated as outpatients. We believe that this minimizes expense to the patient and maximizes quality of remaining life.

Although adenocarcinoma is by far the most common malignant tumor of the pancreas, others do exist and occasionally come to the attention of the ultrasonographer. Perhaps the most common of these is the malignant form of cystadenoma. On ultrasonography, this is usually seen to be a large, septated, fluid-filled lesion that can occur in any segment of the gland but has a predilection for the tail (28–31). Except for the presence of obvious metastatic disease, there is no way of distinguishing the benign from the malignant form of this disorder by ultrasonography. Not all cystadenocarcinomas will have this typical appearance. Some lesions will appear as large, apparently solid masses, and the characteristic cysts will be seen only on microscope examination. Some pathologists, in fact, refer to these as "microcystic adenomas."

Islet cell tumors of the pancreas have no distinctive ultrasonic features (32). Since they often produce distressing metabolic and endocrine changes, such lesions are usually quite small when the patient presents. As a result, they are difficult to diagnose by any of the existing noninvasive techniques. Variable results are reported using selective pancreatic angiography, because islet cell tumors may be associated with considerable hypervascularity.

REFERENCES

1. Mackie C, Bowie J, Cooper M, et al: Ultrasonography and tumor associated antigens. Arch Surg 114: 889–892, 1979.
2. Johnson M, Mack L: Ultrasonic evaluation of the pancreas. Gastrointest Radiol 3: 257–266, 1978.
3. Inamoto K, Yamazaki H, Kuwata K, et al: Computed tomography of carcinoma of the pancreatic head. Gastrointest Radiol 6: 343–347, 1981.
4. Otto R, Deyhle P: Guided puncture under real-time sonographic control. Radiology 134: 784–785, 1980.
5. Buonocore E, Skipper G: Steerable real-time sonographically guided needle biopsy. AJR 136: 387–392, 1981.
6. Bree R, Schwab R: Contribution of mesenteric fat to unsatisfactory abdominal and pelvic ultrasonography. Radiology 140: 773–776, 1981.
7. Crade M, Taylor K, Rosenfield A: Water distention of the gut in the evaluation of the pancreas by ultrasound. AJR 131: 348–349, 1978.
8. Warren P, Garrett W, Kossoff G: The liquid filled stomach: an ultrasonic window to the upper abdomen. J Clin Ultrasound 6: 315–320, 1978.
9. Gooding G, Laing F: Rapid water infusion: a technique in the ultrasonic discrimination of the gas free stomach from a mass in the pancreatic tail. Gastrointest Radiol 4: 139–141, 1979.
10. MacMahon H, Bowie J, Beezhold C: Erect scanning of pancreas using a gastric window. AJR 132: 587–591, 1979.
11. Goldstein H, Katragadda: Prone view ultrasonography for pancreatic tail neoplasms. AJR 131: 231–234, 1978.
12. Meire H, Farrant R: Pancreatic ultrasound—a systematic approach to scanning technique. Br J Radiol 52: 562–567, 1979.
13. de Graaff C, Taylor K, Simonds B, et al: Gray scale echography of the pancreas. Radiology 129: 157–161, 1978.

14. Filly R, London S: The normal pancreas: acoustic characteristics and frequency of imaging. J Clin Ultrasound 7: 121–124, 1979.

15. Marks W, Filly R, Callen P: Ultrasonic evaluation of normal pancreatic echogenicity and its relationship to fat deposition. Radiology 137: 475–479, 1980.

16. Patel S, Bellon E, Haaga J, et al: Fat replacement of the exocrine pancreas. AJR 135: 843–845, 1980.

17. Wright C, Maklad F, Rosenthal S: Grey-scale ultrasonic characteristics of carcinoma of the pancreas. Br J Radiol 52: 281–288, 1979.

18. Weinstein D, Wolfman N, Weinstein B: Ultrasonic characteristics of pancreatic tumors. Gastrointest Radiol 4: 245–251, 1979.

19. Lawson T: Sensitivity of pancreatic ultrasonography in the detection of pancreatic disease. Radiology 128: 733–736, 1978.

20. Pollock D, Taylor K: Ultrasound scanning in patients with clinical suspicion of pancreatic cancer: a retrospective study. Cancer 47: 1662, 1981.

21. Mackie C, Bowie J, Cooper M, et al: Prospective evaluation of gray scale ultrasonography in the diagnosis of pancreas cancer. Am J Surg 136: 575–581, 1978.

22. Taylor K, Buchin P, Viscomi G, et al: Ultrasonographic scanning of the pancreas: prospective study of clinical results. Radiology 138: 211–213, 1981.

23. Gosink B, Leopold G: The dilated pancreatic duct: ultrasonic evaluation. Radiology 126: 475–478, 1978.

24. Weinstein D, Weinstein B: Ultrasonic demonstration of the pancreatic duct: an analysis of 41 cases. Radiology 130: 729–734, 1979.

25. Mitty H, Efremidis S, Yeh H: Impact of fine-needle biopsy on management of patients with carcinoma of the pancreas. AJR 137: 1119–1121, 1981.

26. Ohto M, Saotome N, Saisho H, et al: Real-time sonography of the pancreatic duct. AJR 134: 647–652, 1980.

27. Makuuchi M, Bandai Y, Ito T, et al: Ultrasonically guided percutaneous transhepatic bile drainage. Radiology 136: 165–169, 1980.

28. Carroll B, Sample W: Pancreatic cystadenocarcinoma: CT body scan and gray scale ultrasound appearance. AJR 131: 339–341, 1978.

29. Wolfman N, Ramquist N, Karstaedt N: Cystic neoplasms of the pancreas: CT and sonography. AJR 138: 37–41, 1982.

30. Taft D, Freeny P: Cystic neoplasms of the pancreas. Am J Surg 142: 30–35, 1981.

31. Freeny P, Weinstein C, Taft D, et al: Cystic neoplasms of the pancreas: new angiographic and ultrasonographic findings. AJR 131: 795–802, 1978.

32. Gold J, Rosenfield A, Sostman D, et al: Nonfunctioning islet cell tumors of the pancreas: radiographic and ultrasonographic appearances in two cases. AJR 131: 715–717, 1978.

12

ULTRASONIC DIAGNOSIS OF PANCREATIC CANCER BY REAL-TIME LINEAR-ARRAY EXAMINATION

Tsugio Kitamura

In spite of recent advances in diagnostic investigations for pancreatic cancer, this disease usually is detected too late for cure. If it were possible to perform superselective angiography and endoscopic retrograde pancreatography more easily, pancreatic cancer could be diagnosed in a curable stage. However, because these diagnostic methods require skillful diagnosticians and discomfort for the patient, they often are not carried out. Most patients are not seen until they show relatively obvious signs of pancreatic cancer. The few seen who are in the curative stage are almost without specific symptoms.

Linear-array echography is easily performed and with the improved equipment now available the pancreas can be examined in fine detail (1, 2). In this chapter I will describe results that indicate that this method may permit mass screening and precise diagnosis of early pancreatic cancer.

EXAMINATION TECHNIQUE

An initial longitudinal midline scan is used to establish the level of the pancreatic body. The difference between the levels of the two sides of the pancreas is observed by tilting the transducer to either side. The angle of the longitudinal pancreas for each particular subject is ascertained from true transverse scans. Once the level of the pancreatic body and the angle of the longitudinal axis of the pancreas have been established, transverse scans are performed. In these scans, the above-mentioned angle is revised to display the longest view of the splenic vein. The splenic vein originates from the splenic hilum and crosses over the superior mesenteric artery. At its terminus, it is joined by the superior mesenteric vein to form the portal vein. This knob-shaped point of confluence generally is the widest portion. Because the splenic vein runs close to the upper margin of and directly behind the pancreas, this procedure

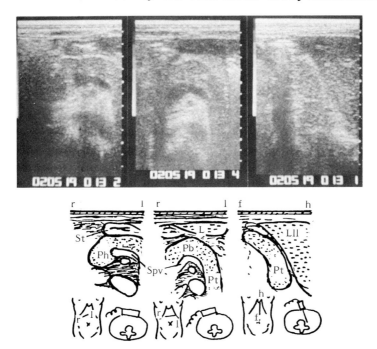

Figure 1.   Linear-array examination of the pancreatic head and tail. (*Left*) For imaging the tail of the pancreas, the left side of the transversely applied transducer is more tightly pressed against the abdomen than the right side. (*Center*) For imaging the tail of the pancreas, the right side of the transversely applied transducer is more tightly pressed against the abdomen than the left side. (*Right*) To image the tail of the pancreas, the longitudinally applied transducer is tilted slightly to the left.

is followed by a slight shift of the scanning plane toward the feet by a tilting or shifting of the transducer.

This procedure allows good visualization of the pancreatic body. Unfortunately, however, the images of the head and the tail are sometimes poor because of obstruction due to gas in the stomach. Compression of the abdominal wall by the transducer is fairly effective in overcoming this. A major advantage of the linear-array transducer is that it makes it possible to scan with the abdominal wall in a compressed state. With the contact compound scanner, when the transducer is pressed against the abdominal wall, it is impossible to scan smoothly, because the transducer depresses the abdominal wall and sinks into the depression.

[1] *Abbreviations used in the figures*: Ao, aorta; Bpd, branches of pancreatic duct; C, cyst; Ca, cancer; Cbd, common bile duct; D, duodenum; f, foot; Gb, gallbladder; h, head; Ivc, inferior vena cava; I, left; L, liver; Li, large intestine; Lll, left liver lobe; Lrv, left renal vein; Mpd, main pancreatic duct; P, pancreas; Pb, Pancreatic body; Pd, pancreatic duct; Ph, pancreatic head; Pt, pancreatic tail; r, right; Rk, right kidney; Rll, right liver lobe; Rra, right renal artery; Rrv, right renal vein; Sma, superior mesenteric artery; Smv, superior mesenteric vein; Spv, splenic vein; St, stomach; T, tumor.

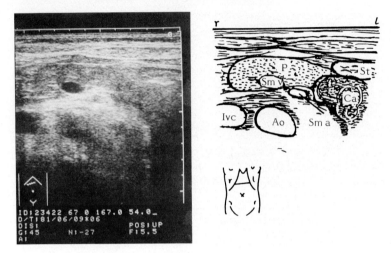

Figure 2. Pancreatic cancer. By pressing the right side of the transducer more tightly to the abdomen, the tumor of the pancreatic tail is more clearly revealed.

The abdominal compression method has the following advantages. First, it can bring the transducer closer to a deep organ such as the pancreas, providing a clear image. Second, it displaces the gaseous contents of the stomach or the intestine. In visualizing the head or tail of the pancreas, the most effective procedure is to press one side of the transducer more tightly against the abdomen than the other. In this way the image of the organ is less disturbed by gastroenteric gas or the costal arch.

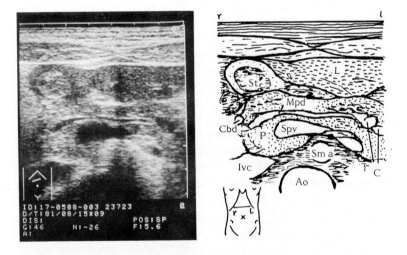

Figure 3. Small cysts of the pancreatic tail. If a dilated pancreatic duct is recognized, it should be followed to where the dilatation ends. In this case it was also necessary to continuously shift the transducer along the dilated pancreatic duct to obtain a correct diagnosis.

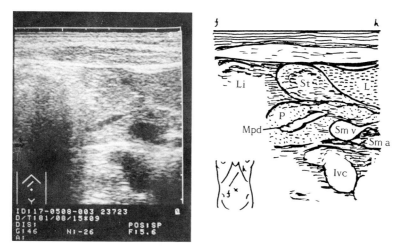

Figure 4.   Dilated pancreatic duct (same case as Figure 3). This sonogram was recorded after the procedure mentioned in Figure 6. The left side of this figure represents the caudal side of the patient and the right side of the figure corresponds to the cranial side of the patient.

The head and the tail of the pancreas can also be visualized by longitudinal or sagittal scanning. By careful tilting the transducer to the right or the left, the head or the tail of the pancreas may be observed together with the pancreatic body. The uncinate lobe is imaged in the right paraspinal region and the pancreatic tail on the left. By scanning the posterial renal region, both parts of the pancreas can be visualized in front of the right or left kidney. Because of the increased attenuation, these scans are not as clear as abdominal scans, and sometimes it is difficult to identify the pancreatic head or tail. The above-mentioned scanning method allows the identification to be made on the basis of their continuity with the image of the pancreatic body. To identify the pancreatic head, one can use the image of the pancreatic part of the common bile duct or the dynamic image of the duodenum as landmarks. The latter can be observed only by real-time scanning (Figures 1–4).

PRESENTATION OF THE ABDOMINAL SONOGRAM

Echograms obtained with real-time equipment may be difficult to interpret because of the variety of scanning planes that can be used. One is able to select any position the patient may assume and scan from any place on the body surface that can accommodate the transducer. For this reason, it is important that scanning data should be presented on the sonogram. Without this data, the echogram not only will be difficult to interpret, but may even lead to a serious misdiagnosis. To facilitate interpretation, diagrammatic rather than direct alphanumeric representation should be employed, because the latter will blot out critical parts of the sonogram.

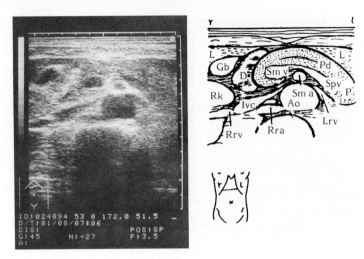

Figure 5. Transverse scanning echogram. In this type of scan the left side of the echogram is the right side of the patient, which is the usual way of presentation.

It is desirable that a diagrammatic illustration accompany the sonogram. It is also useful to include a legend to complement the incomplete representation in the echogram.

In making a correct diagnosis of pancreatic or biliary disease, it is most important to perform serial observation of the pancreatic head region. In this region, the pancreatic duct becomes a common channel with the distal common bile duct or runs longitudinally parallel to the common bile duct. If a dilated main pancreatic duct of the pancreatic body is detected, it should be followed to the end of the dilated pancreatic duct. In such cases the distal portion of the pancreatic duct is usually imaged on the left side of the echogram in the transverse scan. The scanning plane should be shifted from the transverse

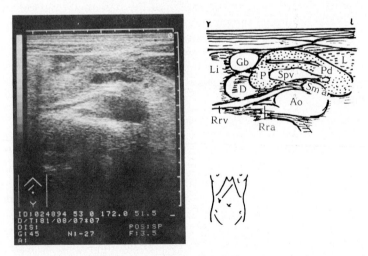

Figure 6. Right subcostal scanning echogram obtained by continuously tracking the main pancreatic duct to the distal portion seen in Figure 5.

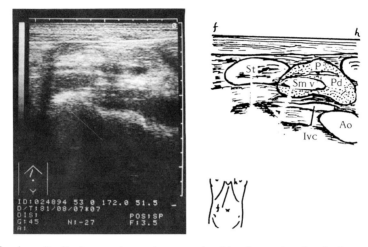

Figure 7. Longitudinal scanning echogram. In this almost longitudinal scan, the left side of the echogram represents the caudal side of the patient. This scan was performed to preserve the continuity of the pancreatic duct in the image.

direction to the longitudinal direction along the course of the main pancreatic duct, so as not to reverse the direction of flow of the pancreatic juice. The caudal portion of the patient will then be imaged on the left side of the echogram. This method is better than examining in the opposite direction to the right side of the patient (3). If the latter method is used, the direction of flow of the pancreatic juice becomes the opposite in transverse scans and this may lead to a serious misdiagnosis (Figures 5–7).

ULTRASONIC SCREENING FOR EARLY PANCREATIC CANCER

Three ultrasonic criteria are available for the diagnosis of early pancreatic cancer: dilated biliary system, enlarged pancreas and swollen spleen. The image of a dilated biliary system suggests cancer of the pancreatic head. The biliary system can be dilated in any of its parts. In the case of a tumor in the pancreatic head, the whole biliary system will appear dilated as far as the common bile duct. Therefore, examination must go beyond the easily detect-

TABLE 1. Biliary Tract Dilatation and Splenic Swelling in Cases of Pancreatic Cancer

Ultrasonic Finding		Biliary Dilatation (positive cases/inspected cases)		Splenic Swelling	
Resected (12 cases)	<3 cm (4 cases)	4/4	(100%)	1/4	(25%)
	>3 cm (8 cases)	4/8	(50%)	3/8	(36%)
Nonresected (38 cases)		21/35	(60%)	17/29	(57%)
Total (50 cases)		29/47	(62%)	21/47	(51%)

TABLE 2. Biliary Dilatation in Cases of Pancreatic Cancer without Jaundice

Cancerous Region	Number of Cases	Dilated Biliary Tract (positive cases/inspected cases)
Head	8	4/8
Head and body	7	1/6
Body	7	2/7
Body and tail	5	0/4
Tail	1	1/1
Total	28	8/26

able dilated gallbladder. Even when a dilated gallbladder is recognized in patients with other disease such as gallstones, chronic liver disease and diabetes mellitus or in patients whose stomach has been operated on, it still can be an important clue to a tumor in the pancreatic head. Whenever an enlarged gallbladder is found, one should also check whether the common bile duct is also dilated. When it is, the pancreatic head region should be surveyed carefully.

The image of a dilated main pancreatic duct also is a clue to early pancreatic cancer, as is an enlarged pancreas itself. Great pancreatic enlargement is indicative of acute pancreatitis or advanced pancreatic cancer, whereas slight enlargement is a clue to early pancreatic cancer.

The last criterion is splenic swelling. If splenic swelling is observed and is not due to hematologic or hepatic diseases, it suggests cancer of the pancreatic body or tail.

The reliability of these criteria was investigated in 50 patients with pancreatic cancer. The cancer in each case was diagnosed histologically by laparatomy. Of the 50 tumors, 12 were extirpated curatively. In the remaining 38

TABLE 3. Sequential Effect of Secrepan on Dilatation of the Main Pancreatic Duct

Minutes after Injection	Number of Cases		Observed Cases	Percent of Effectiveness
	Effective	Total		
5	18	18	47	38.3
10	33	51	64	79.7
15	8	59	73	80.8
20	5	64	72	88.9
25	7	71	80	88.8
30	5	76	82	92.7
35	2	78	79	98.7
Total	87	87	102	76.5

TABLE 4. Sequential Effect of Secrepan on Detection of Branches of the Pancreatic Duct

Minutes after Injection	Number of Cases		Observed Cases	Percent of Effectiveness
	Effective	Total		
0*	10	10	102	9.8
5	7	17	54	31.5
10	19	36	76	47.4
15	16	52	87	59.8
20	6	58	76	76.3
25	9	67	83	80.7
30	2	69	74	93.2
53	1	70	76	92.1
Total	70	70	102	68.6

* In 10 cases, branches of the pancreatic duct had already been observed before the injection of Secrepan.

cases, operations were noncurative or for diagnosis only. In the patients in whom curative surgery was performed, the diameter of the tumor was less than 3 cm in four and greater than 3 cm in eight. As Table 1 shows, innocent swelling of the spleen was not often seen, especially in the extirpated group. It occured in only 25% of patients with tumors less than 3 cm in diameter, suggesting that it is not useful in detecting early pancreatic cancer. It should be noted though that this relatively small group was composed of patients with cancer of the pancreatic head, and the evidence gained from it does not indicate that splenic swelling should be neglected as a clue for detecting cancer of the pancreatic tail. Dilatation of the biliary tract, on the other hand, proved to be of considerable use in detecting early pancreatic cancer (Table 1).

Although dilation of the pancreatic duct is more frequently the direct result of cancer of the head of the pancreas, dilatation of the biliary tract is more easily detected and even anicteric cases of cancer of the pancreatic head reveal dilatation of the biliary tract. Of four anicteric cases of pancreatic cancer, the tumor in two was less than 3 cm and was curatively resected. This data is noteworthy for the diagnosis of early pancreatic cancer (Table 2).

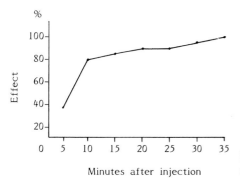

Figure 8. Sequential effect of Secrepan on dilatation of the main pancreatic duct.

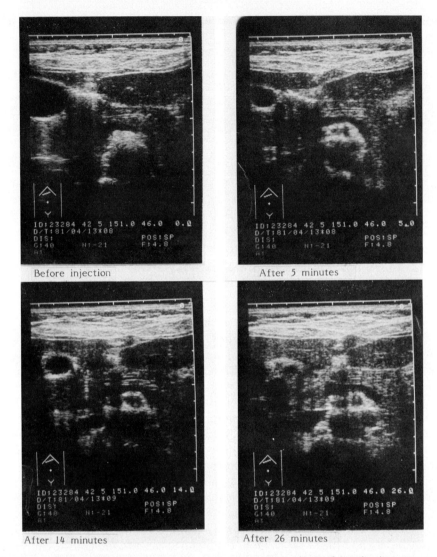

Before injection   After 5 minutes

After 14 minutes   After 26 minutes

Figure 9. Sequential aspects of the main pancreatic duct after the intramuscular injection of Secrepan.

SECREPAN[2]-INJECTION METHOD FOR THE DIAGNOSIS OF PANCREATIC CANCER

Cancer of the pancreatic head or body often causes dilatation of the caudal main pancreatic duct, and this sign can be used in the detection of early pancreatic cancer (4, 6). These dilated pancreatic ducts are not irregular as are

---

[2] Secrepan: preparation for intramuscular injection. One ampule of Secrepan contains 50 units of secretin, a polypeptide extracted from the upper small intestinal mucosal membrane of pig (Eisai Co., Ltd., Japan).

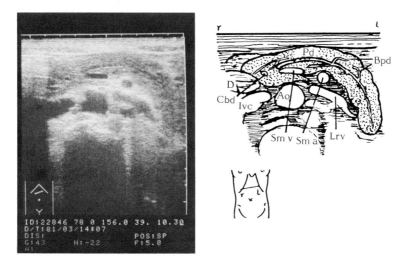

Figure 10.   Branches of the pancreatic duct 10.5 minutes after the intramuscular injection of Secrepan.

those seen in chronic pancreatitis. When the stricture caused by the cancer is not advanced, dilatation of the caudal main pancreatic duct will be absent or very slight. In these cases, injection of drugs that stimulate pancreatic excretion often is effective in clearing the stricture of the pancreatic duct caused by a relatively small tumor. Secrepan injected intramuscularly may be used for this purpose. The most appropriate time for the observation of pancreatic

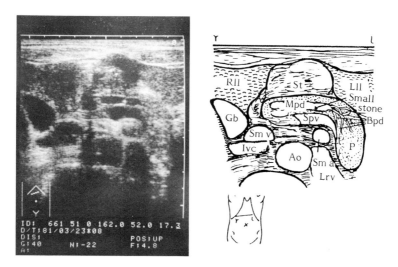

Figure 11.   Chronic pancreatitis 17.5 minutes after the intramuscular injection of Secrepan. The main duct of the pancreatic head and body is dilated and contains a small stone. Several dilated branches are confluent with main pancreatic duct from the pancreatic tail.

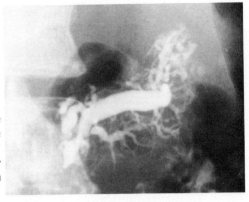

Figure 12. Endoscopic retrograde pancretogram (same case as Figure 10). The findings shown in this figure, except for the small stone, are similar to those revealed in the echogram shown in Fig. 10.

duct dilatation, as shown by the data in Table 3 and Figure 8, is 10–15 minutes after injection (Figure 9). Intramuscular injection of Secrepan also allows visualization of the branches of the pancreatic duct (Table 4, Figures 10–12). The excreted pancreatic juice remains in the duodenum and is also delineated. This is useful in the ultrasonic diagnosis of tumor in Vater's papilla.

It is generally thought that early pancreatic cancer appears ultrasonographically as an irregularly or lobularly outlined mass (7). Many such masses, however, are in fact advanced cancer, and if such a tumor is detected, curative surgery will not always be indicated. The echogram of relatively early pancreatic cancer shows a small tumor with smooth outlines, and the internal echoes of the tumor are of low amplitude and homogeneous (Figure 13).

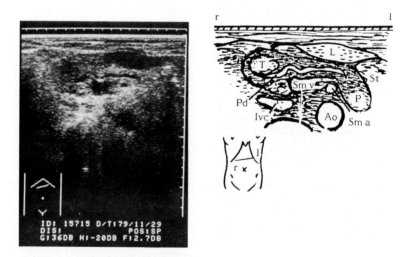

Figure 13. Cancer of the pancreatic head without jaundice. The tumor was resectable. This figure is composed of two continuous echograms.

SUMMARY

In this chapter methods for delineation of the head and tail of the pancreas are described and suggestions with regard to presentation of echograms are given.

In ultrasonic screening for pancreatic cancer, dilation of the biliary tract is a reliable sign, especially in cases of cancer of the pancreatic head. Splenic enlargement also cannot be neglected in detection of cancer of the pancreatic head. Small, resectable pancreatic tumors have smooth margins and homogeneous, low-level internal echoes.

Secrepan injection can clear a stricture of the pancreatic duct, making it possible to detect comparatively small pancreatic tumors. Pancreatic duct dilatation is imaged 10–15 minutes after the injection, whereas branches of the pancreatic duct are best imaged 25–30 minutes later. This method also allows observation of the duodenum.

REFERENCES

1. Kitamura T: Linear Electronic Scanning in Abdominal Ultrasonodiagnosis. Tokyo, Ishiyaku Publisher, 1980.

2. Kitamura T: Guidebook of Abdominal Linear Electronic Scanning. Tokyo, Syuujyunsya, 1981.

3. AIUM standard presentation and labeling of ultrasound images adapted as an interim standard on August 3, 1976. J Clin Ultrasound 4: 393–398, 1976.

4. Ohto M, Saotome N, Saisho H, et al: Real-time sonography of the pancreatic duct: application to percutaneous pancreatic ductography. Am J Roentgenol 134: 647–652, 1980.

5. Parulekar SG: Ultrasonic evaluation of the pancreatic duct. J Clin Ultrasound 8: 457–463, 1980.

6. Oka M, Nishii T, Sakurai T, et al: Evaluation of ultrasonic echodiagnosis of cholelithiasis and cancers of the bile duct and pancreas. Jpn J Surg 1: 42–53, 1971.

7. Meire HB: Differential diagnosis of pancreatic masses. In Hill CR, McCready VR, Cosgrove DO (eds.): Ultrasound in Tumour Diagnosis. Tunbridge Wells, Pitman Medical Publishers, 1978, p 128–144.

13

LIQUID-FILLED STOMACH IN THE ULTRASONOGRAPHIC ASSESSMENT OF THE UPPER ABDOMEN

Peter S. Warren

Richard H. Picker

The stomach and small bowel are dynamic structures that can vary in capacity, shape and location with both intrinsic changes and changes in the surrounding viscera. Any contained gas and unrecognizable solid matter impairs the ultrasonic assessment of the upper abdomen and, as a consequence, when a patient is not examined under relatively standardized conditions, such as fasting and with the proximal gastrointestinal tract filled with liquid (1, 2), difficulty may be experienced in the assessment of those patients suspected of having upper abdominal tumor or in whom the presence of a tumor is known but for whom further information on location and tumor type are sought.

When the stomach is distended with liquid, the relations to it of some normal upper abdominal structures change to accommodate it, and if the patient is examined sitting, erect or prone any gas present rises to the fundus (3). The liver is displaced to the right and rotated counterclockwise, and the colon and distal small bowel are displaced away from the area being studied. The liquid-filled stomach and proximal small bowel then provide:

1) an anatomical landmark,
2) an acoustic window to deeper structures, particularly the stomach bed, and
3) a means for demonstrating the stomach wall.

An acoustic window can be provided by many liquids. Flavored water, orange juice, pineapple juice and tomato juice all are acceptable. Apple juice promotes intestinal peristalsis and is not recommended. The best results, particularly in demonstrating the stomach wall, have been obtained with fruit-flavored 1% methylcellulose aqueous suspension, which allows good through-transmission

176

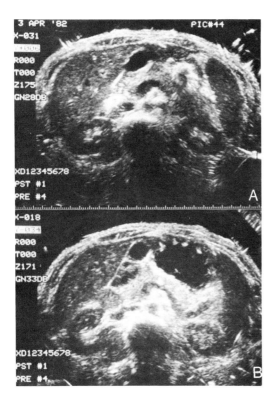

Figure 1. Transverse compound echograms of the upper abdomen at the level of the splenic vein before (A) and after (B) the ingestion of 1 liter of flavored water. The stomach and duodenum are now precisely located and a more satisfactory window to the structures in the stomach bed has been acquired.

of sound and contains inert mucilages that are stable in both alkaline and acid solutions and in the presence of small concentrations of most electrolytes. Compared with water, relatively little air is swallowed with methylcellulose.

The patient is encouraged to drink 1 liter of liquid after fasting overnight and having the procedure carefully explained. It is helpful if the patient is presented with only one or two glasses of liquid at a time rather than being confronted with the total volume initially. Also, it is important that the liquid be taken slowly over half an hour or so to minimize the ingestion of air and to enable the liquid to reach the jejunum. The examination can be performed

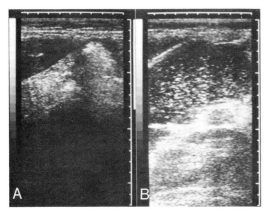

Figure 2. Parasagittal linear-array real-time echograms through the left lobe of the liver before (A) and after (B) the ingestion of 1 liter of flavored water. Gas in the stomach has been displaced by the liquid, creating a window to the left kidney and the body of the pancreas immediately anterior to it. The impression on the posterior wall of the stomach is a reliable localizing sign for the body of the pancreas.

quite satisfactorily without the use of drugs to relax the bowel because, in the absence of gastroenterostomy or other stomach drainage operation, sufficient liquid remains in the stomach for well over an hour after ingestion. Generally all but the sickest patients are able to comply.

Adequate and relatively rapid assessment of the upper abdomen can be performed with real-time scanners, both linear array and sector, when the upper gastrointestinal tract is filled with liquid. Although particularly useful, these scanners generally lack the ability of static scanners to provide both a panoramic view of the upper abdomen and high-quality sequential echograms for a comprehensive retrospective assessment of tumor involvement.

THE VALUE OF THE LANDMARK

When filled with liquid the stomach can be precisely located (Figures 1, 2, 4–6, 13, 14) and its size and shape (Figures 5, 3A, 14), with the saccular proximal and tubular distal parts, readily appreciated. In transverse sections the contours of the distended normal stomach are rounded, often with some flattening of the posterior surface in its middle third where it lies anterior to the left kidney and pancreas. Longitudinal sections usually reveal an impression on the posterior surface of the stomach produced by the body and tail of the pancreas (Figure 3A) but other indentations may be associated with abnormal

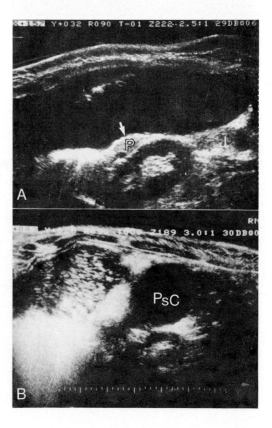

Figure 3. Parasagittal compound echograms of the left upper abdominal quadrant. (*A*) Panoramic section demonstrating the ultrasonic window to the stomach bed in a normal subject created by the liquid-filled stomach. The pancreas (P) returns echoes of slightly higher amplitude than the jejunum (J) from which it is readily distinguished by the location of the accompanying splenic vessels and by the impression on the posterior contour of the stomach (arrow). (*B*) Pancreatic pseudocyst (PsC) in the inframesocolic compartment of the peritoneal cavity inferior to the gas-containing transverse colon and stomach filled with orange juice. High-amplitude echoes are returned from the particulate matter in the orange juice.

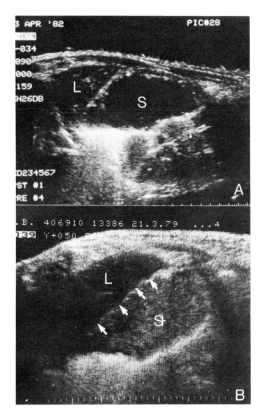

Figure 4. Parasagittal sections through the left lobe of the liver (L) after the ingestion of 1 liter of flavored water. The smooth inferior surface of the normal liver (A) is enhanced by the liquid-filled stomach (S). Liver metastases from colonic carcinoma (B) protruding from the inferior liver surface can be readily recognized (arrows) and are not hidden by the "bloom" often produced by stomach gas.

masses (Figure 5). The anterior surface and lesser curvature of the distended stomach are closely applied to the posteroinferior surface of the left lobe of the liver, which is usually smooth, and any irregularities produced by tumor tissue, particularly multiple metastases, are highlighted, irrespective of the texture of the underlying abnormality (Figure 4).

Filling the duodenum with liquid establishes its location (Figures 1, 8, 11) and its relationship to the gallbladder and to structures in the porta hepatis

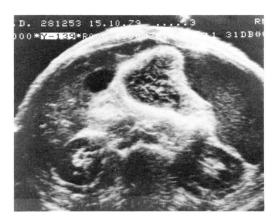

Figure 5. Transverse compound echograms at the level of the renal hila showing the stomach, distended with orange juice. The stomach shows medial displacement and a smooth inward deformity of the greater curvature produced by splenomegaly due to leukemic infiltration.

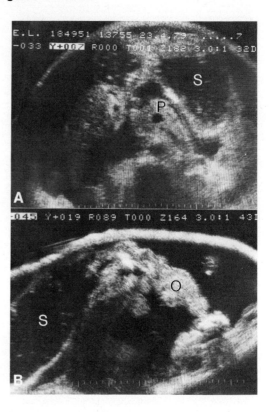

Figure 6. Ovarian carcinoma with gross ascites. (A) Transverse section at the level of the pancreas (P) demonstrating liquid in the greater sac of the peritoneal cavity surrounding the liver and also demonstrating liquid in the inferior recess of the lesser sac between the pancreas and the liquid-filled stomach (S). (B) Parasagittal compound scan through the left side of the abdomen demonstrating a thickened tumor-infiltrated greater omentum (O) attached to the greater curvature of the liquid-filled stomach (S).

(Figure 7). Also, liquid in the second part of the duodenum enables the right border of the pancreatic head to be accurately delineated and avoids the occasional problem of an empty duodenum wrapped around the pancreatic head simulating a pancreatic mass (Figures 1, 8, 11).

When the gastrointestinal tract is filled with liquid, the proximal jejunum can be seen, in longitudinal sections through the left upper quadrant, to be tucked under the root of the transverse mesocolon inferior to the pancreas, without producing an impression on the posterior surface of the stomach. The echoes returned from the jejunum vary in amplitude, depending on its contents, but are usually of lower amplitude than those from the pancreas. The location of the transverse mesocolon can be demonstrated between the stomach and the jejunum and this, together with the demonstration of colonic gas, enables a mass to be assigned either a supramesocolic or inframesocolic location (Figure 3B). The proximal jejunum, when filled with slurry, may be mistaken for the pancreas by the unwary, particularly in transverse sections, and, likewise, liquid at the duodenojejunal flexure may simulate a pancreatic pseudocyst. The correct location of the liquid is ascertained both by observation of the ingestion of liquid and of peristalsis with the real-time scanner.

By the demonstration of the position of the transverse mesocolon, a supramesocolic or inframesocolic location can also be given to liquid collections in the peritoneal cavity. Liquid in the lesser sac may be demonstrated behind the lesser omentum, and, when in the inferior recess, liquid can be seen anterior to the pancreas and posterior to the liquid-filled stomach (Figure 6).

GASTROINTESTINAL TRACT AS WINDOW

The liquid-filled stomach provides an ultrasonic window to the stomach bed by displacing the transverse colon and small bowel inferiorly and displacing the liver slightly to the right. The impression on the posterior surface of the stomach is a very reliable sign for locating the body and tail of the pancreas, and the window enables the pancreas to be demonstrated in its entirety, though not always in a single section, from its right border (seen either through the first part of the duodenum or the liquid-filled gastric outflow tract) out to the region of the hilum of the spleen, accompanied by the splenic vessels (Figures 1–3, 6, 10). The liquid in the stomach provides good through-transmission, allowing less gain to be used for optimal demonstration of the pancreas and, particularly, of the pancreatic duct, which with careful scanning may often be seen throughout its length (Figure 8). The left kidney, which is often best portrayed in coronal scans through the left flank, may also be well demonstrated together with the left renal artery and vein in both transverse and parasagittal sections (Figures 1, 3, 5, 8). The distal duodenum and proximal jejunum are also seen through the window, and their delineation sometimes enables the inferior mesenteric artery to be demonstrated as it passes up behind the proximal jejunum to join the splenic vein 3 or 4 cm lateral to its confluence with the superior mesenteric vein.

The small bowel may also provide a useful acoustic window, particularly to the region of the porta hepatis and bile duct (Figure 7).

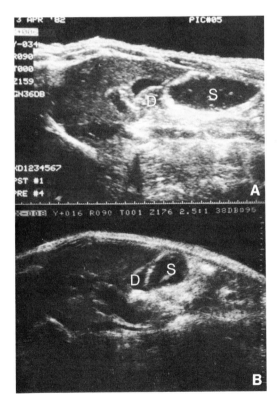

Figure 7. Sagittal echograms through the upper abdomen at the level of the inferior vena cava. The liquid-filled distal stomach (S) and first part of the duodenum (D) act as both a landmark and a window in each case. (*A*) Normal subject showing the relationship of the duodenum to the gallbladder. (*B*) Section through the bile duct (B) in a patient with obstructive jaundice due to an ampullary tumor. The displacement of gas from the stomach and first part of the duodenum facilitates location of the obstruction.

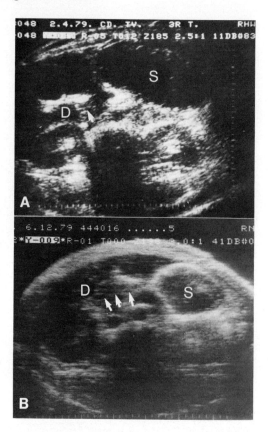

Figure 8. Transverse compound scans at the level of the pancreatic head in two patients in whom the stomach (S) and proximal small bowel (D) have been filled with liquid. The right border of the pancreas is well defined. A normal pancreatic duct (arrow) is seen entering the second part of the duodenum in *A.* In *B* a carcinoma of the head of the pancreas involving the ampulla is demonstrated as a localized area of decreased reflectivity producing distortion and dilatation of the pancreatic duct (arrows) in the head of the pancreas.

Bowel gas in the central abdomen may make it difficult to demonstrate a clinically suspected mass in this region, but if the patient drinks 2 or 3 liters of liquid in the 12 hours before examination, the small bowel may fill with liquid and displace the gas, providing an effective window to the area of interest (Figure 9).

Figure 9. Medial ectopia of the right kidney. Sagittal echogram through the abdomen in a 9-year-old girl in whom a central abdominal mass was felt and in whom a right kidney could not be demonstrated in a normal location by excretion urography. After ingestion of 2 liters of liquid over 12 hours, the liquid-containing small bowel (B), from which most gas has been displaced, provided an excellent window to reveal the true nature of the mass. (S) Stomach.

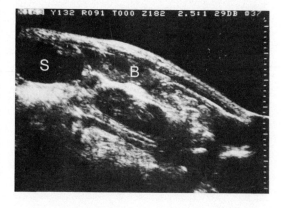

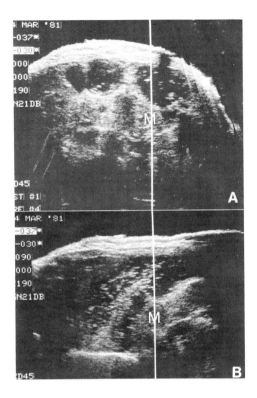

Figure 10. Carcinoma of the body of the pancreas seen through the acoustic window provided by the liquid-filled stomach. Transverse (*A*) and parasagittal (*B*) sections marked with the point of rotation through the localized area of decreased reflectivity (M) in the body of the pancreas. The tumor does not involve the stomach wall.

When the major upper abdominal anatomical landmarks are ultrasonographically visible, recognition and appreciation of the extent of abnormal masses are facilitated (Figures 11–13).

WALL OF THE GASTROINTESTINAL TRACT

When filled with liquid the wall of the stomach and proximal duodenum becomes effaced, aiding the demonstration of the relatively low-amplitude-echo-

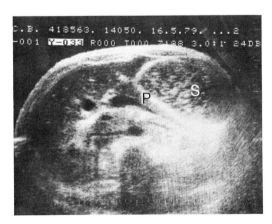

Figure 11. Transverse echogram at the level of the right renal artery in a patient with massive infiltration of the retroperitoneum by lymphoma. The demonstration of the extent of the infiltration on the left side is aided by the acoustic window through the liquid-filled stomach (S). (P) Pancreas.

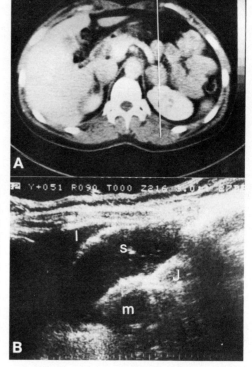

Figure 12. Bilateral adrenal tumors are demonstrated in a computerized tomography scan (a) of the abdomen at the level of the left renal vein. The marker passes through the left adrenal tumor. The ultrasonic window provided by the liquid-filled stomach (S) reveals the adrenal tumor (m) deep to the pancreas in a parasagittal compound echogram of the left upper quadrant. The tip of the left lobe of the liver (l) and the proximal jejunum (J) have also been demonstrated.

producing muscular layers sandwiched between the echogenic mucosa and mucus on the inner surface and the serosa on the outer (Figure 7A) (4). The thickness of the stomach wall may be readily ascertained (Figure 6), and it can be determined whether the stomach wall is involved in a stomach tumor (Figure 13) or in an underlying tumor (Figure 10). When a stomach fails to distend with liquid, is thick-walled and lacks the normal rounded contours, an infiltrative process such as "linitis plastica" (Figure 14) can be strongly suspected. The duodenal wall (Figure 7) and sometimes that of the transverse colon can be seen, allowing some mural abnormalities to be recognized.

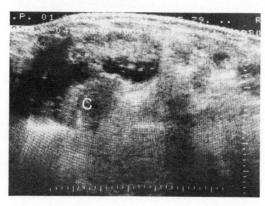

Figure 13. Gastric carcinoma (C). The tumor can be seen passing through the stomach wall into the lesser sac to invade the pancreas in this parasagittal scan through the stomach filled with tomato juice.

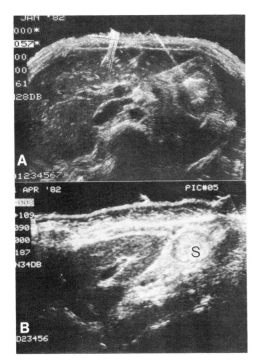

Figure 14. Linitis plastica. The small stomach, which could not be distended with liquid, is seen in the transverse echogram (*A*) at the level of the origin of the left renal vein. The stomach wall is grossly thickened with diffuse infiltration of adenocarcinoma cells. A sagittal section at the level of the aorta in a normal subject (*B*) shows a normal gastric outflow tract (S) with a wall of normal thickness for comparison. The high-amplitude echoes in the lumen are returned from food residues mixed with the ingested liquid.

CONCLUSION

Filling the stomach, duodenum and proximal jejunum with a known liquid in a fasting patient standardizes the anatomy and creates an ultrasonic window to deeper structures. Both real-time and static B-mode scanners can be used with the technique that aids in the recognition and more complete assessment of an abdominal tumor.

REFERENCES

1. Warren PS, Garrett WJ, Kossoff G: The liquid-filled stomach—an ultrasonic window to the upper abdomen. J Clin Ultrasound 6: 315–320, 1978.
2. Crade M, Taylor KJW, Rosenfield AT: Water distention of the gut in the evaluation of pancreas by ultrasound. Am J Roentgenol 131: 227–230, 1978.
3. MacMahon H, Bowie JD, Bezhold C: Erect scanning of pancreas using gastric window. Am J Roentgenol 132: 587–591, 1979.
4. Picker RH, Kossoff G, Warren PS: The use of ultrasound in intrinsic gastric disease—a preliminary report. In Kurjak A (ed): Recent Advances in Ultrasound Diagnosis 2. Excerpta Medica International Congress Series 498. Amsterdam, Excerpta Medica, 1980, pp 374–377.

14

INTRALUMINAL SCANNING: USE OF THE ECHOENDOSCOPE AND ECHOLAPAROSCOPE IN THE DIAGNOSIS OF INTRAABDOMINAL CANCER

Morimichi Fukuda

Ultrasonic examination of the abdominal organs not infrequently suffers from inadequate imaging due to intervening bowel gas and interference with resolution caused by abdominal wall structures. This has been a particularly serious problem in patients with suspected pancreatic diseases. In such cases, the frequency of inadequate visualization of the pancreas, especially of the tail and a portion of the head and of the papillary region, is high.

Intraluminal scanning can alleviate this problem, and in this chapter a short review of the subject will be followed by a description of some of our experience with echoendoscope and echolaparoscope examinations.

HISTORY

The first attempt at ultrasonic intraluminal scanning was made in 1957 by Wild and Reid (1), who used a rotating scan head in the rectum to detect echo pattern changes due to cancer of the rectum. At that time, analyses also were made of the A-mode patterns in colonic and gastric mucosa to elucidate changes characteristic of malignant transformation of these hollow organs.

Unfortunately, a full account of the clinical application of this technique was not provided until some time later, when Japanese investigators, Watanabe et al (2), began to use a specially designed "chair" for the detection of prostatic cancer by radial scanning of the prostate from the rectal lumen.

This technique also was applied to investigation of the female pelvic organs and of the urinary bladder. In the latter, direct introduction of the scanner via the cystocope also met with considerable success (3, 4).

Successful application of intraluminal scanning of the upper abdomen was delayed for some time because of the difficulty of introducing a scanning head safely into the stomach or duodenum through the esophagus. Successful introduction of the ultrasonic scanner into the esophagus was achieved by Japanese workers, Hisanaga and Hisanaga (5), who obtained a B-mode image of the heart. In the United States, Green of SRI International (6) and members of the Mayo Clinic also introduced the use of an electronic linear-array scanner mounted on a gastrofiberscope. The real-time images they obtained from canine stomachs were impressive both in resolution and in grey scaling. Stimulated by this pioneering work, a number of commercial firms have begun the manufacture of such instruments.

ELECTRONIC LINEAR-ARRAY ECHOENDOSCOPE

This apparatus was introduced by DiMango et al (7) of the Mayo Clinic and Green of SRI International. A commercially available side-viewing gastroscope (American Corp. Medical Instruments Model FX-5) was modified by attaching an ultrasonic probe to the end of the endoscope, so that both the optics and the ultrasound were on the same side. The resulting rigid part of the scope was 80 mm long and 13 mm in diameter. The ultrasonic system generated a real-time ultrasonic image with a 10-MHz 64-element linear array that produced a real-time image 3 cm wide and 4 cm deep. An ultrasonic lens and dynamic focusing in both transmission and reception of ultrasound were incorporated, and a digital scan converter was used for image development. Because the apparatus had a rather long, hard tip, human experiments were not performed. Animal experiments via the stomach yielded high-quality echograms of the stomach wall, the liver, the kidney, the large vessels and the pancreas. Intrathoracic scanning through the esophageal wall also resulted in excellent tomograms of the heart and large vessels.

Recently, some Japanese investigators have reported the use of a similar electronic linear-array scanner mounted on the tip of a gastrofiberscope. The resolution and stability of the images were rather inferior because of the use of a lower frequency of 3.5 MHz and a limited field of view. At present, instruments of this type are used primarily for the investigation of intrathoracic lesions, its limited field of view being the major limitation on its use in abdominal investigations.

TRANSESOPHAGEAL RADIAL SCANNER

The development and use of this apparatus was reported by Hisanaga and Hisanaga and by Green et al in the same year. In the beginning this instrument did not employ fiberoptics. It consisted of a small transducer (2.25 or 3.5 MHz), a flexible tube, a flexible rotation shaft in the tube, a potentiometer, a variable-speed motor and a gear-and-lever system. The small transducer inserted into the esophagus was rotated at a rate of 4–15 cycles per second, and the image

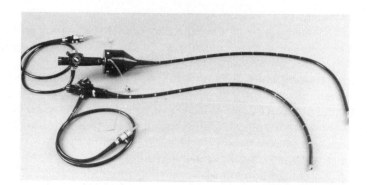

Figure 1. Echoendoscope prototype 1 as compared with a regular gastrofiberscope.

on the cathode ray tube was displayed at the rate of 8–30 fields per second. Good images were obtained from various parts of the heart, but the resolution of the image was somewhat limited by the frequency of the transducer. This apparatus was further improved by adding a fiberscope, and with this instrument the same group of workers obtained images of the intraabdominal organs via the gastric wall as well as of intrathoracic tissues.

Due to the rapid development of echoendoscopes, efforts were made by endoscope manufacturers to develop prototype equipment to be used in routine clinical practice. The first prototype of an echoendoscope that became available was the mirror-type echoendoscope, codeveloped by Olympus and Aloka Co. (Figures 1 and 2). The commercially available fiberscope, Olympus B3 (side-viewing type), was modified by attaching a scanning compartment to the tip of the scope. Scanning was carried out by rotation of the flexible shaft to which the mirror in the scanning head was attached, the shaft being driven by a

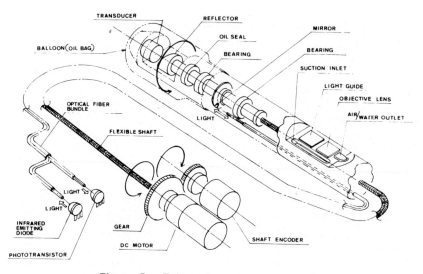

Figure 2. Echoendoscope prototype 1.

small DC motor in the proximal end of the scope. The rotating angle of the mirror, by which an ultrasonic beam from the small transducer fixed at the end of the scope was transmitted to the plane perpendicular to the axis of the scope, was detected by a photosensing mechanism that used infrared light transmitted by fine glass fiber bundles incorporated into the shaft of the scope. The scanning angle was 90°, and relatively good images were obtained. Figures 3 and 4 show echograms of the gastric wall, malignant gastric tumors and images of the pancreas.

The major limitation of the equipment was the rather inferior resolution of the echograms as compared with that of echograms obtained from outside the abdominal wall using a high-resolution real-time scanner with a liquid-filled stomach as an acoustic window. Slight vibration of the image due to uneven rotation of the scanning mirror, which often occurred at the time of strong flexion of the scope, also caused some difficulty in obtaining high-resolution images.

The second prototype of the device, which became available approximately 1 year later, had marked improvements in the scope and the scanning mech-

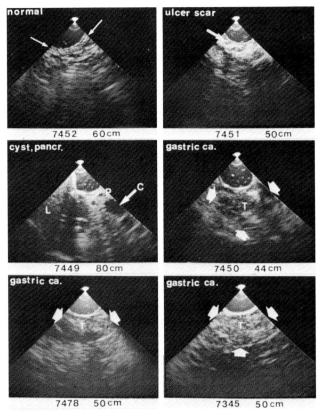

Figure 3. Sector scanning images of the normal stomach, ulcer scar, small pancreatic cyst and three cases of gastric carcinoma (balloon method). L, liver; P, pancreas; C, Cyst; T, gastric cancer.

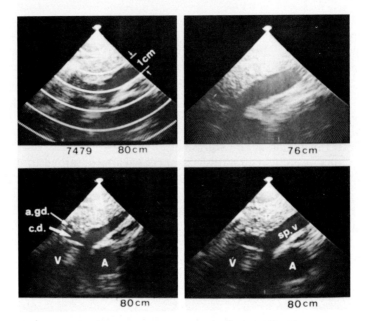

Figure 4. Sector scanning images of the normal pancreas recorded by the echoendoscope, prototype 1. A, aorta; V, inferior vena cava; a. gd., A. gastroduodenalis; c.d., common duct; sp. v, splenic vein.

anisms. Major changes were the use of a small transducer with increased frequency and the adoption of direct rotation of the transducer connected to the flexible shaft. This brought about an increased scanning angle of 180° and a shortening of the rigid part of the scope, which made it feasible to introduce the scanning head safely into the gastric as well as the duodenal lumen (Figures 5 and 6).

The use of a balloon to cover the scanning head and to facilitate the contact of the head with the gastric wall was discontinued. Instead, after routine en-

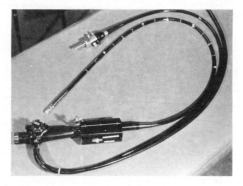

Figure 5. Echoendoscope prototype 2, the transducer rotation type. The 7.5-MHz transducer housed in the tip compartment is 7 mm in diameter. A 180° field is secured.

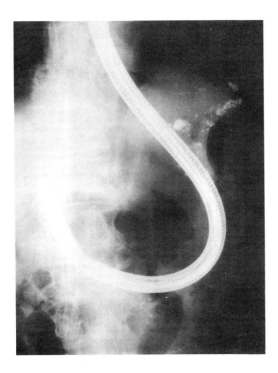

Figure 6. Radiograph showing the scanning head of the echoendoscope in the first portion of the duodenum.

doscopic observation by the same fiberscope, deaerated water was introduced into the gastric or duodenal lumen through the thin corrugation channel prepared in the shaft of the scope. This technique, another liquid-filled stomach method, had never been employed in gastric echography because of the suspected danger of erroneously aspirating the gastric contents into the airway during examination. However, no such accidents were experienced during 50 examinations, and no complaints were heard from patients. The only precautions necessary were the use of a goodly amount of Xylocaine jelly to anesthetize the pharynx and careful handling of the scope itself.

It soon became apparent that subtle changes in the mucosa of the gastric wall could not be depicted without the use of the water fill-up method, which naturally distended the wall. Furthermore, organs or lesions in juxtaposition with the gastric wall could never be adequately visualized unless the scanning head was kept some distance (2–3 cm) from the gastric wall to avoid blurring of the image by side lobes. By following these procedures, the resolution of the image became extremely good, as can be seen in Figures 7–12. With surprisingly good resolution, it was possible to identify a small submucosal tumor in the gastric wall that was later identified as an aberrant pancreas (Figures 7 and 8). Malignant as well as benign ulcerations of the stomach, including the extent of gastric wall involvement, were readily diagnosed (Figures 9 and 10). Superb resolution was also obtained from the pancreas (Figures 11 and 12), both in normal and in pathological conditions, over the entire region of the organ. The only necessary maneuver was careful positioning of the patient to guide the scanning head to the desired portion of the stomach wall to be scanned, i.e., the right decubital position for scanning the head of the pancreas

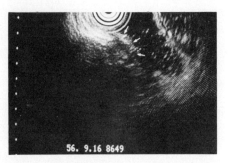

Figure 7. A radial scanning image of a submucosal tumor (arrows) of the stomach, aberrant pancreas, obtained by the echoendoscope, type 2.

and the left decubital position for scanning the body and tail. After guidance of the scanning head was completed, no further movement of the scope was necessary, because respiratory excursion allowed observation of the entire organ.

Comparison of intraluminal scans has clearly shown their superiority to echograms obtained from outside the abdominal wall. This method also is applicable to the examination of other organs, such as the spleen, kidney, adrenal

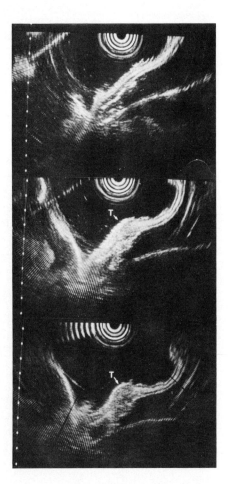

Figure 8. Sonograms of a resected submucosal tumor of the stomach, aberrant pancreas, placed in a water tank. Scanning of the resected specimen by the same echoendoscope clearly showed the presence of a submucosal tumor in the gastric wall. Five layers, the mucosa, submucosa, muscle layer, subserosa and serosal layers, and the tumor are clearly demonstrated. (T)

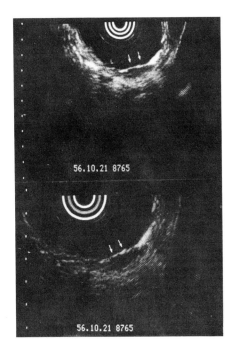

Figure 9. Sonograms of a chronic gastric ulcer of the angulus. Arrows indicate the ulcer, which was covered by a thin layer of fibrin. The nonechoic layer underneath represents granulation tissue of the ulcer.

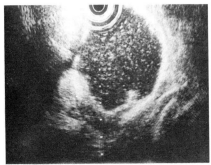

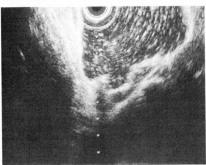

Figure 10. Sonograms of a malignant gastric ulcer obtained from a patient with ulceration in the center of well-demarcated gastric carcinoma.

193

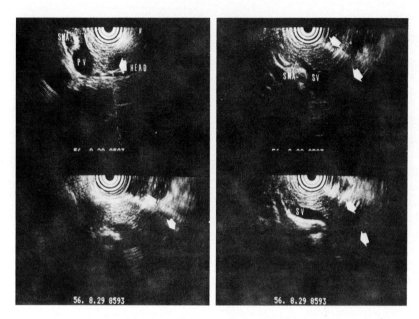

Figure 11. Echograms of the normal pancreas recorded by the echoendoscope. Arrows indicate the head of the pancreas. PV, portal vein; SMA, superior mesenteric artery; SV, splenic vein.

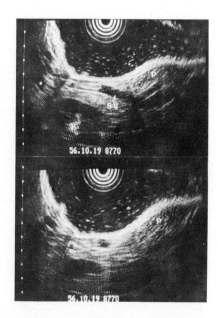

Figure 12. Sonograms of the tail of the pancreas recorded by the liquid-filled stomach method. Parenchymal tissue (p) of the pancreatic tail was well demonstrated beneath the stretched stomach wall. Part of the left kidney and splenic vein (SV) are shown.

glands, gallbladder and liver. Although the instrument has not yet been tested for use in the lower digestive tract, on the basis of the quality of the images obtained so far, it seems safe to say that the method will prove to be well suited for the survey of malignant changes in the lower colon and the rectum.

ECHOLAPAROSCOPY

The use of echography during laparoscopic examination was first attempted by Japanese investigators, Yamakawa and Wagai (10). As early as 1958, Wagai had detected some characteristic echo patterns of gallbladder cancer using A-mode scanning under laparoscopic guidance. Due to the invasiveness of the technique and to limited diagnostic information, this type of examination was soon discontinued until recently, when the endoscope manufacturer Olympus developed the first prototype of the echolaparoscope. The first reports on the clinical use of the system were made in 1981 and further details were presented at the 4th European Congress on Ultrasonics in Medicine in Dubrovnik in the same year (11).

At present, two types of equipment are available (Figure 13). The apparatus consists of an ordinary laparoscope with a scanning compartment, in which a small transducer and a reflecting mirror are housed in an arrangement similar to that employed in the first prototype of the echoendoscope. The field of view, which corresponds to the plane perpendicular to the axis of the scope, is 90°. The transducers used are 7.5 and 10 MHz and 7 mm in diameter.

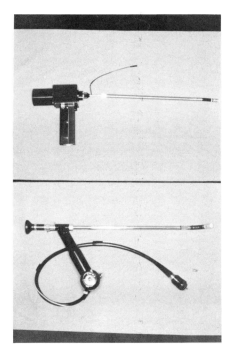

Figure 13. The first and second prototype echolaparoscope. The details of the second, the Olympus A 5211, are as follows: external diameter, 10 mm; view angle, 70°; length, scanner, 24 mm; flexible part, 35 mm; total length, 334.5 mm; angle of flexion, 110°; frequency, 7.5 MHz; scan mode radial scan (Mirror); diameter, transducer, 7 mm; focus range, ~30 mm; scan angle, 90°.

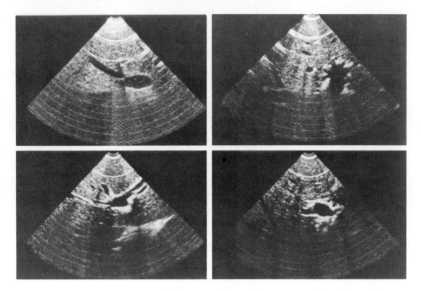

Figure 14. Sonograms of the normal liver obtained with the echolaparoscope, type 1. Numerous fine tributaries of the portal veins are well demonstrated as are branches of the hepatic veins.

After routine laparoscopic examination, the scanning laparoscope was introduced into the abdominal cavity through the trocar and the scanning head was gently placed on the surface of the organ to be examined. The reflecting mirror in the scanning compartment was rotated by a DC motor housed in the pistol-type grip on the other end of the scope or by a motor in a small, separate

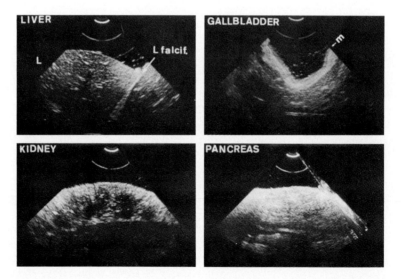

Figure 15. Sonograms recorded by in vitro scanning of human organs obtained from a cadaver. Very fine details are described in the respective organs by the 10-MHZ (Megahertz) transducer.

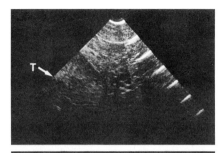

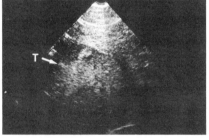

Figure 16. Sonograms of primary hepato-cellular carcinoma obtained by scanning with the echolaparoscope equipped with a 10-MHz transducer. Fine details of the tumor nodule are easily recognized, even though attenuation of the sonic wave is considerable. T, tumor.

motor box that was connected to the scope by a flexible shaft similar to that used in the echoendoscope. The resulting ultrasonic images displayed on a digital scan converter screen were either directly photographed or stored on videotape.

The images obtained by the echolaparoscope, especially those obtained with the 10-MHz scanning head, were of excellent quality. They allowed observation not only of the minute tributaries of the intrahepatic vasculatures but also of the circulating blood, swirling in the portal vein stem (Figure 14).

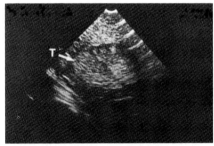

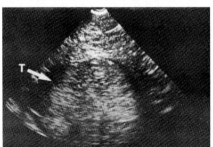

Figure 17. Sonograms recorded from the patient whose sonograms are shown in Figure 16. At a frequency of 7.5 MHz, good penetration is obtained. T, tumor.

Scans of the human organs obtained at the time of necropsy are shown in Figure 15. As is apparent, resolution was superb. The three-layer structure of the gallbladder wall, the fine tributaries of vessels in the liver, the papillary structure in the pelvis of the kidney and the characteristic echo patterns of the pancreas all could be observed.

A clinical survey of the liver in which this instrument was used showed that with it observations could be made that were not possible by sonographic examination from outside the abdominal wall. Occult lesions in the liver, such as metastatic deposits, primary hepatocellular carcinoma and cysts could be visualized without difficulty. In cases of hepatocellular carcinoma in particular, sonolaparoscopic examination disclosed very fine details of tissue changes characteristic of primary hepatoma, such as the nodules in the nodule sign, septas, capsules and even some abnormal vessels in the tumor.

The sonolaparoscope can also be used to guide biopsy of hidden lesions in the liver. Although ultrasonic guidance can be used for blind biopsy by the Silverman needle, the danger of bleeding prohibits its routine use. Detection of deeply seated lesions by this technique, followed by biopsy under direct vision, may be the most appropriate use for this invasive technique.

CONCLUSION

Although the discussion in this chapter largely has been confined to the use of the echoendoscope and echolaparoscope for diagnosing upper abdominal diseases, a similar technique should be applicable to lesions of any organ in the abdominal cavity. The use of high-frequency transducers has markedly improved the resolution of ultrasonic images. Although the techniques employed are semiinvasive or invasive, if they are used wisely they can provide crucial diagnostic information.

ACKNOWLEDGMENT

This paper was supported, in part, by a Grant-in-Aid for Cancer Research (54-1) from the Ministry of Health and Welfare of Japan.

REFERENCES

1. Wild JJ, Reid JM: Progress in techniques of soft tissue examination by 15 MC pulsed ultrasound. In Kelly E (ed.): Ultrasound in Biology and Medicine. Washington DC, American Institute of Biological Science, 1957, p 30–45.

2. Watanabe H, Katoh H, Katoh T, et al: Diagnostic application of the ultrasonotomography for the prostate (in Japanese). Jpn J Urol 59: 273–279, 1968.

3. Holm HH, Northeved AA: Transurethral ultrasonic scan. J Urol 111: 238, 1974.

4. Niijima T: Ultrasonic diagnosis and bladder cancer staging. In Wagai T, Omoto R (eds): International Conference Series 505.

5. Hisanaga K, Hisanaga A: A new real-time sector scanning system of ultra-wide

angle and real-time recording of entire adult cardiac images: transesophagus and transchest wall methods. In White D, Lyons EA (ed): Ultrasound in Medicine Vol 4. New York, Plenum Press, 1978, pp 391–402.

6. Green PS: Biomedical ultrasonics at SRI International ALUM-JSUM Joint Conference, Dec. 5, 1978, Honolulu, Hawaii. Japan J Med Ultrason 16: 223–229, 1979.

7. DiMagno EP, Buxton JL, Regan PT, et al: Ultrasonic endoscope. Lancet 1: 627–629, 1980.

8. Fukuda M, Hirata K, Saito K, et al: On the diagnostic use of echoendoscope in abdominal diseases. I. Diagnostic experiences with a new type echoendoscope on gastric diseases. Proc Jpn J Med Ultrason 37: 409–410, 1980.

9. Fukuda M, Ohmi N, Terada S, et al: On the diagnostic use of echoendoscope in abdominal diseases. II. Diagnostic experiences with a new model of echoendoscope. Proc Jpn J Med Ultrason 39: 405–406, 1981.

10. Yamakawa K, Wagai T: Diagnosis of intraabdominal lesions by laparoscope. 4. Ultrasonography through laparoscope. Jpn J Gastroent 55: 741, 1958.

11. Fukuda M, Hirata K, Saito K, et al: Studies on intraluminal echography in abdominal disease: echolaparoscopy. In Kurjack A (ed): Proceedings, 4th European Congress on Ultrasonics in Medicine, International Congress Series 547. Amsterdam, Excerpta Medica, 1981, p 109.

15

ULTRASONIC MANIFESTATION OF THE SPLEEN

Takashi Koga

Even today the spleen is an organ of mystery. Although it is assumed to play a role in resistance to infection, hematopoiesis and immunity, few clinicians have paid attention to splenic changes.

Recently, however, many ultrasonic studies have revealed that the spleen changes its size, reflecting various diseases. For example, splenic changes have been observed in viral hepatitis, liver cirrhosis, hepatocellular jaundice, hepatocellular liver carcinoma and systemic malignant neoplasms. Thus, information on splenic changes has proved to be of value not only in the recognition of splenic disease but also of various generalized diseases. Therefore, ultrasonographers should include the spleen in their examinations.

ULTRASONIC MANIFESTATION OF THE SPLEEN

Scanning Procedure

The spleen lies in the left upper quadrant of the abdomen and may be visualized by contact compound transverse or longitudinal scans with the patient in the supine or prone position. Our procedure is as follows: the spleen is scanned parallel to the rib in the IXth intercostal space with the patient in the right decubitus position. The splenotomogram obtained by this scanning method is compatible with the section parallel to the longitudinal axis of the spleen. The section along the longest axis of the spleen is useful in determining change in the size of the spleen.

Qualitative Analysis

Splenotomograms may be classified on the basis of their shape, contour and size, with consideration of internal echogenicity by the method of sensitivity-graded tomogram, as previously described (1, 2).

200

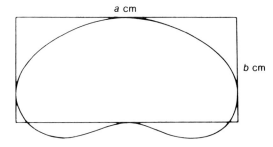

a cm

b cm

Figure 1. Model for simplified calculation of cross-sectional area of spleen.

Quantitative Analysis

The area of the spleen may be used to judge splenic size. Our simplified method for determining this area (S) consists of using the formula $S = k \times R$, where ($R = a \times b$) is the rectangular area of the spleen calculated from its longitudinal length (a) and width (b), as shown in Figure 1. The constant K was 0.8 in normal subjects (100 adults) and 0.9 in 96 patients with liver diseases. In normal individuals, the mean value of the calculated sectional area is about 12 cm^2 and never exceeds 20 cm^2 (1–3).

Numerous methods have been proposed for the determination of spleen volume from several sectional areas of the organ. Our simplified method for calculating spleen volume (4) uses the formula $V = 7.5 \times (S - 10)$, where V is the volume and S the area of the spleen. Figure 2 shows the good linear correlation between area and the volume in 10 removed spleens. The method has also been found useful in clinical practice (4).

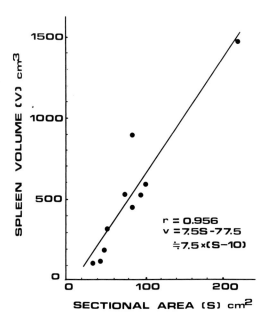

$r = 0.956$
$v = 7.5S - 77.5$
$\doteqdot 7.5 \times (S-10)$

Figure 2. Correlation of area with volume of removed spleens.

TABLE 1.   Ultrasonic Classification of Splenomegaly

Diffuse Homogeneous Splenomegaly
Type I: soft pattern (inflammatory)
    Type I-a (acute inflammatory)
        Acute hepatitis, sepsis, endocarditis, and others
    Type I-b (chronic inflammatory)
        Chronic hepatitis, common cold, rickettsiosis, hypochromic anemia, thrombopenic
        purpura, aplastic anemia, myelofibrosis, cardiac failure, and others
Type II: intermediate pattern (congestive)
    Liver cirrhosis, Banti's syndrome, portal hypertension, hemolytic spherocytosis, ma-
    lignant lymphoma, Hodgkin's disease, myeloma, some Leukemias, and others
Type III: hard pattern (proliferative)
    Chronic myelogenous leukemia, malignant lymphomas

Localized Heterogeneous Splenomegaly
Benign lesions: cyst, hematoma, abscess, infarct, etc.
Malignant lesions: metastatic neoplasms

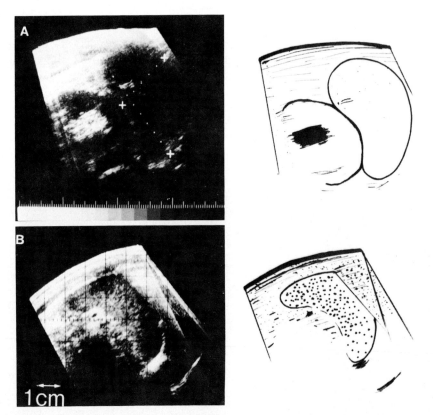

Figure 3.   Type I: soft pattern of splenomegaly. (*A*) Type 1-a. 43-year-old man with acute hepatitis on eighth day after onset of clinical signs. *S* (sectional area), 52.2 cm^2; *Vc* (calculated volume), 317 cm^3. (*B*) Type 1-b. 34-year-old man with chronic hepatitis 6 months after first admission. *S*, 36.7 cm^2; *Vc*, 200 cm^3.

ULTRASONIC CLASSIFICATION OF SPLENOMEGALY

Diffuse homogeneous splenomegaly, except those with localized lesions, can be divided into three types based on ultrasonic tomograms obtained by scanning parallel to the rib (Table 1).

Type I: Soft Pattern

Type I-a (Figure 3a): The anterior edge is round, the margin is indistinct and it generally appears soft. The longitudinal and vertical axes enlarge. A spleen in the initial stages of inflammation shows this pattern. The internal echoes appear highly homogeneous.

Type I-b (Figure 3b): The margin becomes more distinct, indicating a slightly firmer organ. This pattern appears in chronic inflammations, some hematologic diseases, cardiac failure and other diseases.

Type II: Congestive Pattern

This pattern is intermediate between Types I and III. The longitudinal and vertical axes are grossly enlarged, the anterior and posterior splenic angles appear markedly round, with diffuse, internal echoes at a medium level (Figure 4). Congestive spleen in liver cirrhosis shows this pattern.

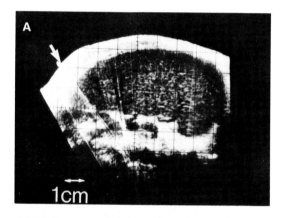

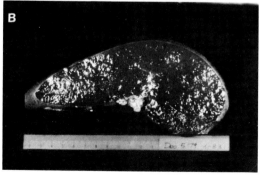

Figure 4. Type II: congestive pattern of splenomegaly. 43-year-old man with liver cirrhosis in stationary phase. Arrow in *a* indicates rib margin. *S*, 212.5 cm^2; *Vc*, 1,516 cm^3. Splenotomogram (*A*) is consistent with section parallel to longest axis of removed spleen (*B*). *V*$_a$ (actual volume of removed spleen), 1,000 cm^3.

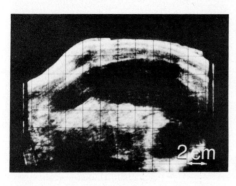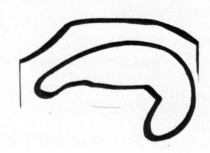

Figure 5.   Type III: hard pattern of splenomegaly. 32-year-old man with chronic myelogenous leukemia in stationary phase. *S*, 104.8 cm^2; *Vc*: 711 cm^3.

Type III: Hard Pattern (Figure 5)

The outline of the spleen is distinct, with a sharply angular anterior edge. The
organ looks hard and extremely enlarged along both axes. The internal echoes
are at the lowest level of the three types. A spleen in the stationary phase of
chronic myelogenous leukemia shows this pattern.

DIFFUSE HOMOGENEOUS SPLENOMEGALY

It has been claimed that malignant neoplasms of the spleen are rare (5, 6).
Recently, several investigators have characterized splenic neoplasms (7–12).

Between 1971 and 1980, we diagnosed only 65 instances of this splenic abnormality, not counting hepatocellular diseases. These spleens were usually
examined by oblique scanning parallel to the ribs to obtain the longitudinal
section along the longest axis of the organ. Of the 65 cases of malignant splenomegaly, 56 showed the diffuse homogeneous patterns listed in Table 1, fall-
ing with equal numbers into one of the three basic patterns (13).

Although it was not always possible to differentiate leukemia from lymphoma, splenotomograms in cases of chronic myelogenous leukemia mostly
showed the typical Type III pattern, whereas those in cases of malignant lymphoma showed mostly Type II, and occasionally Type III, patterns.

Their sectional areas ranged from 20 to 200 cm^2 as shown in Figure 6. The
mean value was 96.2 ± 46.1 cm^2 in 12 cases of chronic myelogenous leukemia
and 87.4 ± 45.4 cm^2 in 10 cases of malignant lymphoma. The spleens in patients with these two diseases were significantly larger than those in patients
with liver cirrhosis. In 33 cases of the latter the mean value was 52.4 ± 20.9
cm^2.

Some of the ultrasonic studies of leukemia and lymphoma, including Hodgkin's disease, have suggested that spleens with infiltrative malignancy produce
a more sonolucent appearance than the enlarged spleen in portal hypertension
(8, 12, 14, 15). The splenotomograms of patients with leukemia display mostly
Type III patterns, as illustrated in Figure 7. The margins are distinct, with
sharply angular anterior edges, and the internal echoes are quite low. The

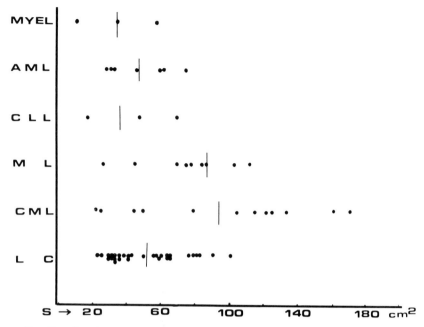

Figure 6. Sectional areas of spleen with leukemia (22), lymphoma (10), myeloma (3) and liver cirrhosis (33). MYEL, myeloma; AML, acute myelogenous leukemia; CLL, chronic lymphogenous leukemia; ML, malignant lymphoma; CML, chronic myelogenous leukemia; LC, liver cirrhosis.

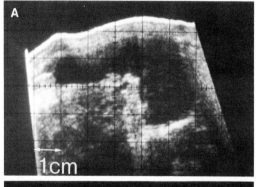

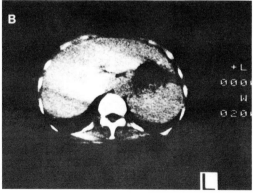

Figure 7. Chronic myelogenous leukemia. 59-year-old woman. (a) S, 37.1 cm², V, 203 cm³. (b) CT 10 cm above the umbilicus. The density of the spleen is lower than that of the liver.

205

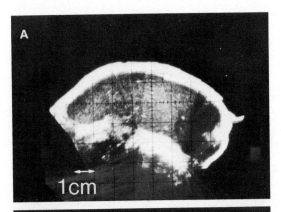

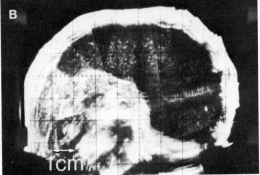

Figure 8. Chronic myelogenous leukemia. 29-year-old man under medical treatment. (*a*) Oblique scan parallel to the ninth rib. Magnification, ⅓. S, 160.7 cm²; V, 1,130 cm³. (*b*) Transverse scan 10 cm above the umbilicus. The enlarged spleen is more sonolucent than the liver.

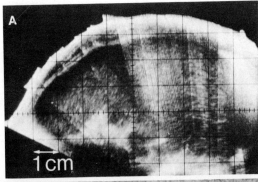

Figure 9. Malignant lymphoma. 76-year-old man with T-cell lymphoma and acute generalized infection. Autopsy was performed on the eighth day after the ultrasonic examination. (*a*) Oblique scan parallel to ninth rib. The high-level echoes from the posterior half are due to air in the lung over the semidiaphragm covering the posterior pole of the spleen. Magnification, ⅓. S, 233.1 cm²; V, 1,671 cm³. (*b*) Gross appearance of the spleen after autopsy. V_a (actual volume), 1,220 cm³.

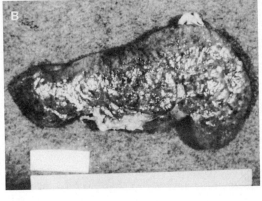

206

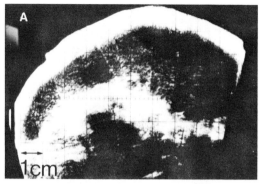

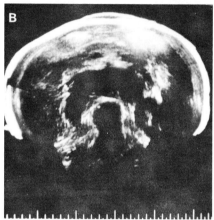

Figure 10. Malignant lymphoma. 25-year-old woman with Hodgkin's disease 3 months before death. (a) Oblique scan parallel to the ninth rib. S, 109.3 cm²; V, 742 cm³. (b) Transverse scan 10 cm above the umbilicus. Markedly enlarged abdominal lymph nodes are present.

splenotomogram shown in Figure 7 shows a hard organ. It was obtained from a patient in a stationary phase of chronic myelogenous leukemia. In a patient with exacerbated chronic myelogenous leukemia, the spleen showed a Type III pattern with a rather high level of internal echoes (Figure 8).

The splenotomograms of patients with lymphoma display mostly Type II patterns (Figure 9). The anterior edge is round, and the internal echoes are rather high, giving the appearance of a rather congested organ. On the other hand, some splenotomograms in patients with Hodgkin's disease show a Type III pattern (Figure 10), whereas the spleen in acute myelogenous leukemia shows mostly a Type I-b pattern. Thus, ultrasonic findings of spleens involved in leukemia or lymphoma depend on the phase and type of disease.

LOCALIZED HETEROGENEOUS SPLENOMEGALY

Benign Lesions

Cyst

Although splenic cysts are much less common than cysts arising in the liver and kidney, it is well known that ultrasound is a most effective tool for their detection (16–20).

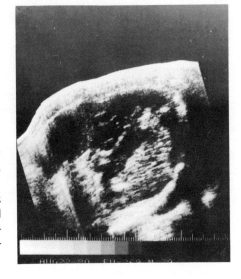

Figure 11. Hematoma due to rupture of spleen. 39-year-old laborer with splenic injury 1.5 months after a landslide accident. The patient suffered fracture of the left eighth, ninth and tenth ribs, and developed left pleural and abdominal hemorrhagic effusion. The diagnosis was confirmed by laparotomy performed 3 months after injury.

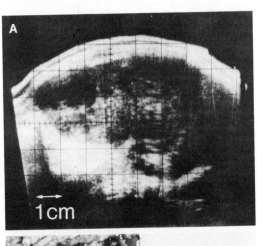

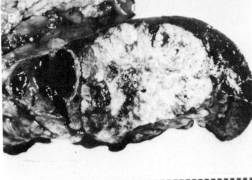

Figure 12. Metastatic melanoma. 57-year-old woman with splenic metastasis of melanoma originating from the nasal mucosa. (A) Splenotomogram parallel to the ninth rib. (B) Gross appearance of cut surface of removed spleen parallel to longest axis.

208

Hematoma (21—23), Abscess (24—26) and
Infarct (27)

These should be distinguished from malignant abnormalities. An example of splenic injury is shown in Figure 11. The enlarged spleen with hemorrhage and hematoma is occupied by low- and high-level echo areas, surrounded by sonolucent pleural and abdominal effusion.

Malignant Lesions

Melanoma

Although several cases of metastatic melanoma in the spleen have been reported (28–31), this localized neoplasm is rare. In our series, there were two instances of localized splenic metastases. One of them is shown in Figure 12. The low-level echo areas at the anterior pole correspond to the necrotic tissue mass and the highest-level areas to the proliferative tumor mass in the removed spleen.

ULTRASONIC PATHOLOGY

In 1968, Kikuchi, one of the pioneers of ultrasonography, coined the term "ultrasonic pathology" and initiated a quantitative method in ultrasonic diagnosis using "sensitivity-graded tomogram pairs" (32). We have employed sensitivity-graded tomography to characterize splenic tissue for the purpose of differential diagnosis of splenic diseases (2). This method is also available to judge localized heterogeneous abnormalities of the spleen. Unfortunately, it is not easy to distinguish among diffuse homogeneous splenomegaly by these methods.

Recently, Kossoff et al (33) described a classification of soft tissues by grey scale echography that has been adopted widely, and Chivers (34) reviewed the published reports on tissue characterization by ultrasonography.

Among ultrasonic investigations of splenic neoplasms, Taylor and Milan (8) reported the differentiation of consistency of splenic tissue by amplitude A-scan analysis, Nicholas (35) described methods for judging tissue characterization by frequency analysis, and Mittelstaedt and Partein (12) emphasized the importance of splenic internal echo density. Indeed, analysis of the internal echogenicity of the spleen is useful in the characterization of the splenic tissue, but it must be taken into account that the tissues may change their reflectivity with the phase and type of the disease and in response to various complications, such as inflammatory infiltration, congestion and malignant cell proliferation. Extensive investigation is needed to establish ultrasonic pathology.

ACKNOWLEDGMENTS

I thank my colleagues for their clinical assistance, Mr. K. Makino for his technical assistance and my wife Sachiko for her secretarial assistance. I also appreciate the encouragement of Prof. A. Sumiyoshi, First Department of Pathology, and Prof. Y. Minamishima, Department of Microbiology, Miyazaki Medical College, who also read the manuscript.

REFERENCES

1. Koga T, Morikawa Y: Ultrasonographic determination of the splenic size and its clinical usefulness in various liver diseases. Radiology 115: 157–161, 1975.
2. Koga T: The spleen. In de Vlieger M (ed): Handbook of Clinical Ultrasound. New York, John Wiley & Sons, 1978, pp 327–333.
3. Petzoldt R, Lutz H, Ehler R, et al: Beurteilung der Milzgrösse mit der Ultraschnittbildmethode. Med Klin 71: 2113–2116, 1967.
4. Koga T: Correlation between sectional area of the spleen by ultrasonic tomography and actual volume of the removed spleen. J Clin Ultrasound 7: 119–120, 1979.
5. Berge T: The metastasis of carcinoma with special reference to the spleen. Acta Path Microbiol Scand Suppl 188: 1–128, 1967.
6. Daniels V, Kummerle F, Preiss J, et al: Die Staging-Laparotomie bei malignen Lymphomen. Dtsch Med Wschr 106: 233–238, 1981.
7. Carlsen EN: Liver, gallbladder and spleen. Radiol Clin North Am 13: 543–556, 1975.
8. Taylor KJW, Milan J: Differential diagnosis of chronic splenomegaly by grey-scale ultrasonography: clinical observation and digital A-scan analysis. Br J Radiol 49: 519–525, 1976.
9. Hunter TB, Haber K: Unusual sonographic appearance of the spleen in a case of myelofibrosis. Am J Roentgenol 128: 138–139, 1977.
10. Weill FS: Ultrasonography of digestive diseases. Saint Louis, The CV Mosby Co, 1978, pp 441–469.
11. de Graeff CS, Taylor KJW, Jacobson P: Grey-scale echography of the spleen follow-up in 67 patients. Ultrasound Med Biol 5: 13–21, 1979.
12. Mittelstaedt CA, Partein CL: Ultrasonic-pathologic classification of splenic abnormalities: grey-scale patterns. Radiology 134: 697–705, 1980.
13. Koga T, Makino K: The ultrasonic tomogram of the spleen XXIII. Pattern and size of malignant splenomegaly. Jpn J Med Ultrasonics 38: 457–458, 1981.
14. Vicary FR, Souhami RL: Ultrasound and Hodgkin's disease of the spleen. Br J Radiol 50: 521–522, 1977.
15. Gless TP, Taylor JW, Gazet JC, et al: Accuracy of grey-scale ultrasonography of liver and spleen in Hodgkin's disease and the other lymphomas compared with isotope scans. Clin Radiol 28: 233–237, 1977.
16. Bhimji SD, Cooperberg PL, Naiman S, et al: Ultrasound diagnosis of splenic cysts. Radiology 122: 787–789, 1977.
17. Popper RA, Weinstein BJ, Skolnick ML, et al: Ultrasonography of hemorrhagic splenic cysts. J Clin Ultrasound 7: 18–20, 1979.
18. Thurber LA, Cooperberg PL, Clement JG, et al: Echogenic fluid: a pitfall in the ultrasonographic diagnosis of cystic lesions. J Clin Ultrasound 7: 273–278, 1979.
19. Glancy JJ: Fluid-filled echogenic epidermoid cyst of the spleen. J Clin Ultrasound 7: 301–302, 1979.

20. Brinkly AA, Lee JKT: Cystic hamartoma of the spleen. CT and sonographic findings. J Clin Ultrasound 9: 136–138, 1981.

21. Kristensen JK, Burmann B, Kuhl E: Ultrasonic scanning in the diagnosis of splenic haematomas. Acta Chir Scand 137: 653–657, 1971.

22. Asher MW, Parvin S, Virgilio RW, et al: Echographic evaluation of splenic injury after blunt trauma. Radiology 118: 411–415, 1976.

23. Cunningham JJ, Wooten W, Cunningham MA: Grey-scale echography of soluble protein and protein aggregate fluid collections (in vitro study). J Clin Ultrasound 4: 417–419, 1976.

24. Brown JJ, Sumner TE, Crowe JE, et al: Preoperative diagnosis of splenic abscess by ultrasonography and radionuclide scanning. South Med J 72: 575–577, 1976.

25. Cunningham JJ: Ultrasonic findings in isolated lymphoma of the spleen simulating splenic abscess. J Clin Ultrasound 6: 412–414, 1978.

26. Grant E, Mertens MA, Mascatello VJ: Splenic abscess. Comparison of four imaging methods. Am J Roentgenol 132: 465–466, 1979.

27. Itoh K, Hayashi A, Kawai T, et al: Echography of splenic infarct in a case of systemic lupus erythematosus. J Clin Ultrasound 6: 113–114, 1978.

28. Shocket E, Dembrow VD: Splenic metastases from a melanoma of the nasal mucosa. Am J Surg 106: 949–953, 1963.

29. Murphy J, Bernardino ME: The sonographic findings of splenic metastases. J Clin Ultrasound 7: 195–197, 1979.

30. Gebel M: Space occupying lesions of the spleen detected by ultrasonography (Abstr). In Second Meeting of The World Federation for Ultrasound in Medicine and Biology, Miyazaki, Japan, p 257, 1979.

31. Altmeyer P, Noedl F, Merkale H: Lymphogene Metastasierungsbereitschaft des malignen Melanomas: eine retrospective Analyse von 202 lymphadenektomierten patienten. Dtsch Med Wschr 105: 1769–1772, 1980.

32. Kikuchi Y: Way to quantitative examination in ultrasonic diagnosis. Med Ultrasonics 6: 1–8, 1968.

33. Kossoff G, Garrett WJ, Carpenter DA, et al: Principles and classification of soft tissues by grey-scale echography. Ultrasound Med Biol 2: 89–105, 1976.

34. Chivers RC: Tissue characterization. Ultrasound Med Biol 7: 1–20, 1981.

35. Nicholas D: Tissue characterization in vivo by ultrasonic backscattering analysis. In Hill Cr, McCready VR, Cosgrove DO (eds): Ultrasound in Tumour Diagnosis. London, Pitman Medical, 1978, pp 258–272.

16

SONOGRAPHIC FEATURES OF KIDNEY, ADRENAL AND BLADDER TUMORS

Robert K. Zeman

Kenneth J. W. Taylor

Arthur T. Rosenfield

Sonography plays a central role in the diagnosis and staging of urinary tract tumors. Herein we will review the sonographic features of renal, adrenal and bladder tumors. Differential diagnosis and the use of other imaging modalities will be considered so that a logical diagnostic approach to urinary tract neoplasms may be formulated.

KIDNEY

Refinements in gray scale ultrasound equipment now allows detailed visualization of normal intrarenal structures. Renal scanning is optimally performed with the patient in the supine and coronal positions, utilizing the liver or spleen as an acoustic window and as a reference for cortical echogenicity. Occasionally, prone scans may be necessary. The normal renal cortex is less echogenic than normal liver or spleen parenchyma (Figure 1) (1, 2). The medulla appears even less echogenic than the cortex. The arcuate vessels give rise to punctate, intense echoes at the corticomedullary junction (2).

Diagnostic Approach

Despite the many advances in cross-sectional imaging, the intravenous urogram remains the basic screening technique for the detection of renal masses. With respect to renal masses, urograms can be classified into five major categories. These include normal, definite cystic mass, definite solid mass, definite mass-nature unknown and possible mass. On the basis of these categories the subsequent evaluation of the patient may be tailored (3).

212

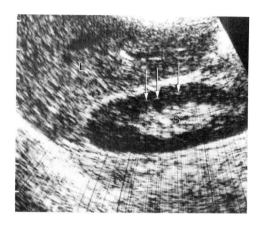

Figure 1. Sagittal sonogram. Normal renal parenchyma is less echogenic than liver (L). Notice the arcuate vessels at the corticomedullary junction (arrows). (S) Renal sinus.

When a possible renal mass is suspected on urography, renal isotope scanning with a cortical agent such as ^{99m}Tc-glucoheptonate or ^{99m}Tc-dimercaptosuccinic acid is recommended. This allows differentiation between real lesions and renal pseudotumors (e.g., septa of Bertin). Pseudotumors typically show normal or slightly increased isotope activity as opposed to tumors that are "cold" (4). Sonography might potentially be of value in this group of patients with possible masses, but theoretically suffers lack of sensitivity because of its tomographic nature and because it cannot take advantage of the fact that pseudotumors contain functioning renal parenchyma.

When a definite renal mass is seen on urography, nephrotomograms will frequently give some indication of the solid or cystic nature of a lesion (5). If a lesion appears cystic or unknown in nature, sonography is carried out to determine whether the lesion represents a simple cyst or other type of mass. If nephrotomography suggests a solid lesion, then staging by one of the cross-sectional techniques is essential. In our preliminary experience (6) computerized tomography is superior to ultrasound in staging, especially in detection of regional and distant nodal metastases. Sonography provides an alternative and relatively accurate method of staging with respect to venous and hepatic abnormalities.

Inasmuch as the majority of renal masses urographically detected are suggestive of cysts, sonography is carried out in the majority of renal masses. Thus, although computerized tomography (CT) is superior in the staging of malignant tumors, ultrasound imaging does obviate the need for CT in a large number of patients. Sonographically, renal masses may appear purely cystic, predominantly solid or complex. It is on the basis of this classification that we present the differential diagnosis of renal tumors.

Ultrasonic Pattern-Purely Cystic

Simple renal cysts are seen in up to 50% of patients over the age of 50. Major criteria are required to be certain one is dealing with a simple cyst (Table I). These criteria are absence of internal echoes excluding artifacts, such as reverberation and "partial volume" effects, sharply defined smooth walls and

TABLE 1.   Renal Cyst

Major Criteria
    Absence of internal echoes
    Sharply defined smooth walls
    Through transmission of beam
Minor Criteria
    Refraction artifact
    Reverberation artifact
    Septation

good transmission of the ultrasound beam so that there is acoustic enhancement of the cyst's back wall (7, 8).

Shadowing from the lateral margins of a cyst due to refraction of the ultrasound beam is seen (9) (Figure 2). Spurious anterior echoes may also be seen within a simple cyst. These are due to reverberation of the ultrasound beam between an anterior reflector and the transducer face. The septae of multiloculated cysts may also produce internal echoes, which can be a source of diagnostic difficulty.

Renal ultrasound is highly accurate in distinguishing a simple cyst from other pathology. Work done before the refinement of gray scale ultrasound established a 90% accuracy in distinguishing cyst from tumor (10). Technical advances have made the current diagnostic accuracy higher. Because of the very high prevalence of renal cysts, we no longer advocate the routine puncture of lesions which meet all the major sonographic criteria for a simple cyst. Localized hydronephrosis, renal artery aneurysms, arteriovenous malformations and hematomas may be purely cystic at times. Therefore, if these lesions are suspected, other uroradiologic studies may be indicated (3). One must be aware that homogeneous tumors such as renal lymphoma, Wilms tumor and melanoma may be echo poor, but they almost never meet all the criteria for a simple cyst on optimal scans (11).

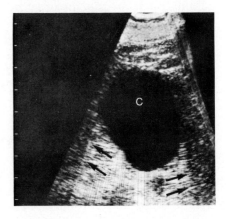

Figure 2. Coronal sonogram. A large left renal cyst (C) shows absence of internal echoes, sharply defined smooth walls and good through transmission of the ultrasound beam. Shadowing (arrows) due to refraction artifact is seen. (Reprinted with permission from CRC Critical Reviews in Diagnostic Imaging, 1981. Copyright, The Chemical Rubber Co., CRC Press, Inc.)

Ultrasonic Pattern-Predominantly Solid

Renal Cell Carcinoma

Renal cell carcinoma accounts for up to 85% of malignancy involving the kidney (12). This tumor typically affects males in the sixth decade with one-third presenting with hematuria and another one-third with a palpable mass. Unfortunately, 20% of patients have no early symptoms referable to their tumor and a late diagnosis may result (12).

Robson's modification of the Flocks and Kadesky staging scheme has gained acceptance because of its correlation between stage and prognosis (13) (Figure 3). The majority of patients present with stage I or II disease, resulting in an at least 60% 5-year survival rate (13). Stage III disease has a significantly worse prognosis largely because of metastatic nodal involvement. Renal vein or inferior vena caval involvement by tumor poses a technical challenge in the operating suite, but probably does not affect long-term survival (14).

Aggressive surgery for patients with stage III or less disease is advocated by many authors (13, 14). Imaging is useful in distinguishing those patients with stage IV disease from the other groups. The surgical approach may be tailored to include a combined thoracoabdominal operation, vena caval resection or even en-bloc lymph node dissection if the extent of tumor is correctly assessed preoperatively. Preoperative arteriography remains a matter of personal preference. Many surgeons feel they need a vascular "road-map" before surgery. Intravenous digital arteriography will increase the availability of this vascular anatomy.

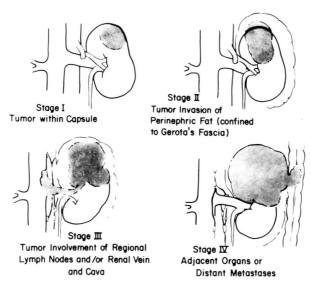

Stage I
Tumor within Capsule

Stage II
Tumor Invasion of
Perinephric Fat (confined
to Gerota's Fascia)

Stage III
Tumor Involvement of Regional
Lymph Nodes and/or Renal Vein
and Cava

Stage IV
Adjacent Organs or
Distant Metastases

Figure 3. Staging of renal cell carcinoma. (Reprinted with permission from CRC Critical Reviews in Diagnostic Imaging, 1981. Copyright, The Chemical Rubber, Co., CRC Press, Inc.)

Sonographically, most renal cell carcinomas are predominantly solid. These tumors usually attenuate the ultrasound beam, have irregular margins and possess variable degrees of internal echogenicity. Hypernephromas as small as 1 cm may be diagnosed, but perhaps not as easily as a cyst of this size (15). Renal cell carcincoma may be more echogenic than, less echogenic than or just as echogenic as renal parenchyma (15, 16). In one series, tumors with echogenicity equal to renal cortex were most common (15). In these patients one must rely on distortion of the renal contour and loss of corticomedullary definition to make the diagnosis (Figure 4). Renal cell carcinoma may appear relatively echo free because of necrosis, hemorrhage or papillary/cystic histology. Subtle low-level internal echoes, irregular margins or attenuation of the ultrasound beam out of proportion to the cystic component of a mass suggests these relatively echo-poor lesions and indicates the need for further studies.

If a solid lesion is detected, extended sonography including the renal vein, inferior vena cava, right atrium, liver and lymph nodes should be performed (17). Direct invasion by tumor of other organs may be present but difficult to identify. The contralateral kidney should also be studied to determine whether metastatic lesions or a synchronous second primary is present. When thrombus is detected in the inferior vena cava (Figure 5), it is usually tumor, but could also represent bland thrombus. The appearance of the thrombus itself is nonspecific. When lymph node involvement is identified, it may be possible to also see vascular compression of the aorta or vena cava (Figure 6).

Transitional Cell Carcinoma

Transitional cell tumors involving the kidney represent 10% of renal neoplasms. The peak incidence is in the seventh decade with a 3:1 male predominance (18). Most tumors of the collecting system are detected as filling defects on intravenous urograms. Clot and stones can mimic tumors at urography. Sonography often can distinguish among these filling defects, and CT also can be used with success in this distinction (19).

Transitional cell carcinoma may contain low-level echoes splitting the normally echogenic renal sinus on sonograms (19) (Figure 7). Advanced transitional cell carcinoma can invade the kidney with total loss of normal renal architecture. Since coexistent thrombosis of the renal vein may be present, severe parenchymal abnormalities may be secondary to venous obstruction rather than direct tumor involvement. Blood clot may produce a mass within the renal sinus similar in appearance to transitional cell carcinoma (Figure 8). Clot, however, should not persist on sequential studies. Stones within the collecting system, if they are large enough, produce an acoustic shadow and therefore can be differentiated from other lesions of the renal pelvis. Small stones may be better evaluated by CT (20). The potential of ultrasound for staging transitional cell lesions of the renal pelvis has yet to be determined.

Wilms Tumor

Wilms tumor is the most common abdominal malignancy of childhood. Ninety percent of children with this disease present with a large palpable flank mass.

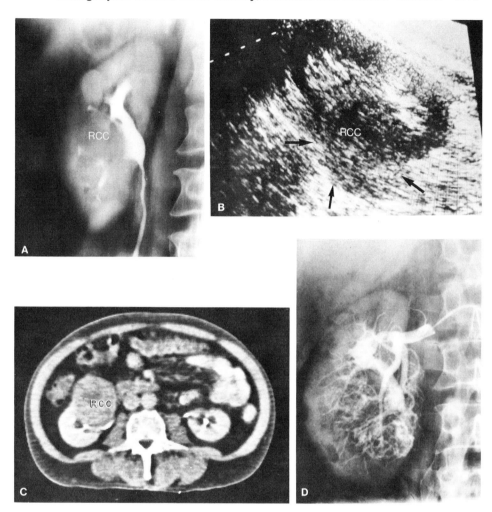

Figure 4. (*A*) Excretory urogram. A large renal cell carcinoma (RCC) is distorting the collecting structures. (*B*) Sagittal sonogram. The tumor (RCC) with its hetero-geneous texture produces an obvious contour deformity of the kidney (arrows). (*C*) CT scan after intravenous injection of contrast medium. Irregular enhancement of the renal cell carcinoma (RCC) is identified. (*D*) Selective right renal arteriogram. A large hypervascular mass compatible with renal cell carcinoma has replaced much of the lower pole. Notice that the echogenicity detected on sonography may not always cor-relate with the degree of tumor vascularity. (Reprinted with permission from CRC Critical Reviews in Diagnostic Imaging, 1981. Copyright, The Chemical Rubber, Co., CRC Press, Inc.)

Areas of internal hemorrhage may give the lesion a deceptively rapid rate of growth. The mean age at presentation is 30 months (21).

Wilms tumors have a variable but usually heterogeneous appearance. There may be multiple small anechoic lucencies within the lesion as well as foci of increased echoes (Figure 9) (22, 23). Cystic degeneration and hemorrhage ap-

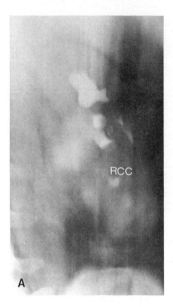
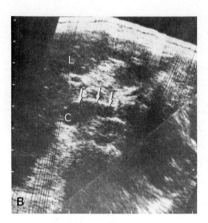

Figure 5. (*A*) Excretory urogram. A left lower pole renal cell carcinoma (RCC) is present. (*B*) Transverse sonogram. Tumor is identified filling the left renal vein (arrows) and protruding into the inferior vena cava (C). (L) Liver.

pear to be responsible for them. Often a hypoechoic rim of compressed renal cortex surrounds the lesion (23).

Once a Wilms tumor is suspected sonographically, an effort should be made to visualize the liver, inferior vena cava, retroperitoneal nodes and the contralateral kidney (23). The incidence of bilateral tumors is at least 5–10% (24). Inasmuch as inferior vena cava involvement by tumor (thrombus) is relatively uncommon, sonography may be acceptable as a screening technique to determine whether an inferior vena cavagram is necessary (23). Once sonography has determined the organ of origin of an abdominal mass and its potential operability, operative biopsy and removal is inevitable. The prognosis in Wilms tumor depends ultimately on histology and surgical staging. Preliminary data suggest that histologic grade is not predicted by the sonographic appearance. Sonography occasionally is helpful in distinguishing postoperative changes from tumor recurrence in the child who has undergone nephrectomy.

The differential diagnosis of Wilms tumor includes neuroblastoma and congenital mesoblastic nephroma. The latter occurs in the neonatal age group and tends to run a benign course. Neuroblastoma can be sonographically identical to Wilms tumor when it invades the kidney, rather than being clearly extrarenal. The presence of tumor calcification with acoustic shadowing is more suggestive of neuroblastoma.

Lymphoma

Although renal involvement with lymphoma is commonly found at autopsy, surprisingly few cases are diagnosed antemortem. Sonography in renal lymphoma usually reveals a relatively echo-poor mass or masses (Figure 10) (11). Adenopathy may be present and possibly produce hydronephrosis. Various patterns of renal involvement, such as multiple renal nodules, direct invasion by perirenal disease, a solitary nodule and diffuse renal infiltration, occur (25). The multinodular form can mimic adult (dominant) polycystic disease (26) on both urography and sonography. Renal involvement with Burkitt lymphoma is being recognized with increasing frequency in the younger patient.

Metastases

Metastases to the kidney are more common than primary tumors but most of these are small and inapparent on imaging studies. The primary tumor in order of decreasing frequency is lung, breast, stomach and pancreas (27). Much as with lymphoma, multiple masses or diffuse renal infiltration help in making the diagnosis, as does a known history of malignancy. Although many me-

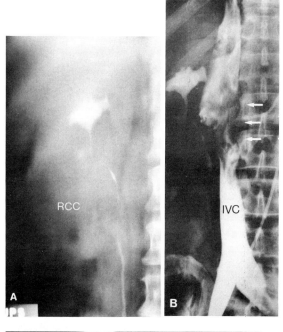

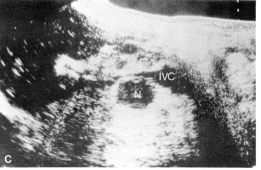

Figure 6. (*A*) Excretory urogram. A right lower pole renal cell carcinoma (RCC) is present. (*B*) Inferior vena cavagram. A long segment of the cava (IVC) is devoid of flow (arrows). This could be due to intrinsic thrombus or flow defect. (*C*) Sagittal sonogram. Enlarged metastatic lymph nodes (N) are seen compressing the posterior aspect of the inferior vena cava (IVC), accounting for the flow defect seen on contrast study. (Reprinted with permission from CRC Critical Reviews in Diagnostic Imaging, 1981. Copyright, The Chemical Rubber, Co., CRC Press, Inc.)

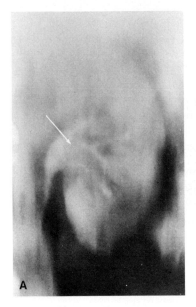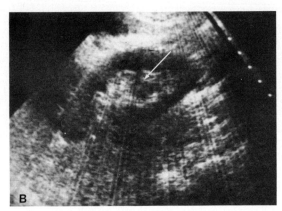

Figure 7. (*A*) Excretory urogram. A filling defect is seen distorting the left renal pelvis (arrow). (*B*) Sagittal sonogram. A lucent mass (arrow) is seen within the renal sinus. Ultimately, this proved to be a 1.5-cm transitional cell carcinoma (courtesy of Dr. John J. Cronan, Providence, Rhode Island).

tastatic lesions are less echogenic than renal cortex, no clear-cut echo pattern based on histology has been established.

Angiomyolipoma

The solitary angiomyolipoma is a lesion most commonly seen in middle-aged women. Pain or hematuria related to hemorrhage is a frequent presenting symptom. The presence of blood vessels, muscle and adipose tissue is responsible for the characteristic sonographic and radiographic appearance of the

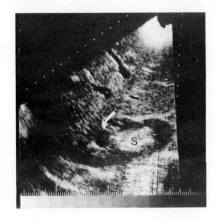

Figure 8. Sagittal sonogram. A lucent mass (arrow) is seen within the upper pole renal sinus (S). This mass resolved and represented clot from recent passage of a renal calculus. It may be difficult at times to distinguish clot from transitional cell carcinoma if follow-up exams to look for resolution are not performed.

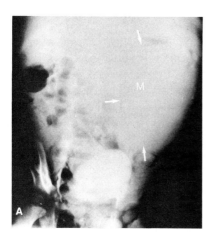
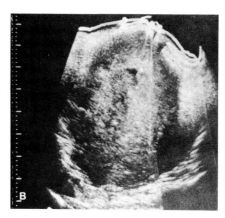

Figure 9. (A) Excretory urogram. A large mass (M) in this child has replaced much of the left flank (arrows). The kidney is destroyed. (B) Transverse sonogram. Wilms tumor with a heterogeneous texture and several areas of necrosis is identified. It may be difficult to determine the organ of origin or render a specific diagnosis in cases such as this.

angiomyolipoma (Figure 11) (28, 29). Echo-free areas within these lesions are usually due to hemorrhage, but areas with relatively less fat can also appear more lucent than other portions of the tumor. The echogenic appearance of these tumors is not specific, but, when these appearances are seen at sonography, CT should be carried out to identify fat and confirm the diagnosis.

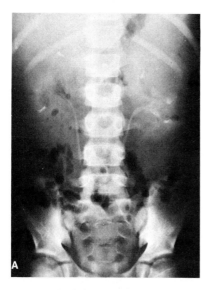
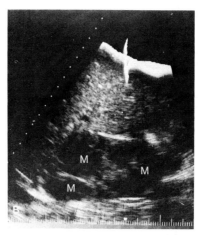

Figure 10. (A) Excretory urogram. Multiple masses within both kidneys distort the collecting systems bilaterally. The spleen is enlarged. (B) Sagittal sonogram. Multiple lucent masses (M) are seen in the right kidney representing Burkitt lymphoma. Note the similarity to polycystic kidney disease. The left kidney was also involved.

Oncocytoma (Renal Tubular Adenoma)

This benign tumor represents a type of cortical adenoma whose existence has been debated in both the radiologic and pathologic literature (30, 31). A rare tumor, it contains oxyphyllic cytoplasm without evidence of cellular atypia. It may be histologically difficult to distinguish from renal cell carcinoma. Its lack of invasiveness and benign course are the ultimate criteria for making the diagnosis.

Sonographically, these lesions are moderately echogenic and of variable size (Figure 12). There should be no evidence of metastatic foci. There is nothing specific about the appearance of an oncocytoma that would allow differentiation from other solid tumors.

Pseudotumors

Pseudotumors are masses of normal renal parenchyma that mimic a pathologic process on urography (32). The subcapsular nodule (so-called splenic bump) also appears as an ultrasonographic pseudotumor because of its moderately echogenic appearance and distortion of the renal contour. The presence of normal corticomedullary definition in the area of contour deformity distinguishes pseudotumors from true lesions. Similarly, areas of focal hypertrophy adjacent to scarring from previous ischemic or inflammatory disease can mimic a mass but should be acoustically identical to normal renal parenchyma. In difficult cases, radioisotope scanning will lead to the correct diagnosis.

Ultrasonic Pattern-Complex

Those lesions that contain largely echo-free internal structures but with definite echogenic foci must be investigated largely on the basis of the clinical setting. Renal abscess, hematoma, hemorrhagic or infected cysts, localized hydronephrosis and cystic nephroma can all appear as complex lesions. Any solid tumor with hemorrhage or necrosis can also appear complex. Although CT and

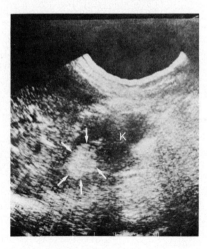

Figure 11. Sagittal sonogram. A highly echogenic mass is seen in the upper pole of the right kidney (arrows). Fat density was identified upon CT, confirming the diagnosis of angiomyolipoma. (K) kidney.

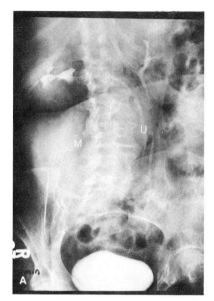

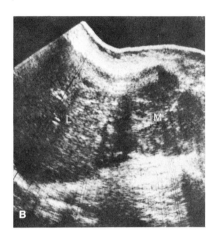

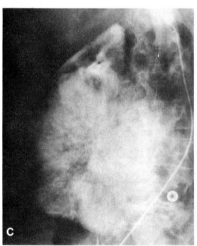

Figure 12. (A) Excretory urogram. Large right renal mass (M) is seen to displace the ureter (U) anteriorly and to the left. (B) Sagittal sonogram. A solid mass (M) filling the midabdomen is present. There is no evidence of metastatic spread. (L) Liver. (C) Right renal arteriogram, capillary phase. The typical "spokewheel" vascular appearance of a renal oncocytoma is visible. The sonographic appearance is nonspecific for this entity.

angiography are both potentially beneficial in evaluating these lesions, liberal use of the 22-gauge "skinny" needle for aspiration of fluid and cytology makes further imaging superfluous in many cases. Although bleeding as a complication is possible when vascular lesions are aspirated, the risk is not significant with small-gauge needles.

ADRENAL GLAND

Sonography of the adrenal gland is technically difficult. Because of this, CT has become the primary screening technique for adrenal pathology at many institutions. Ultrasound may be helpful in very thin patients or in those patients with large palpable masses. Personal expertise and equipment availability will also dictate the choice of modality.

The adrenals are scanned using the liver and spleen as acoustic windows whenever possible. Transverse and coronal scans are performed with the patient in the right lateral decubitus position to visualize the left adrenal. The right adrenal is usually well seen on both coronal and supine transverse scans bordered by the right lobe of the liver, inferior vena cava and right crus of the diaphragm (33). The right adrenal most often has a crescent shape, while the left adrenal is triangular. Enlargement of the gland with bowing of its normally concave margins is indicative of the presence of a mass lesion. Significant enlargement of the right adrenal will produce a posterior impression on the inferior vena cava (Figure 13).

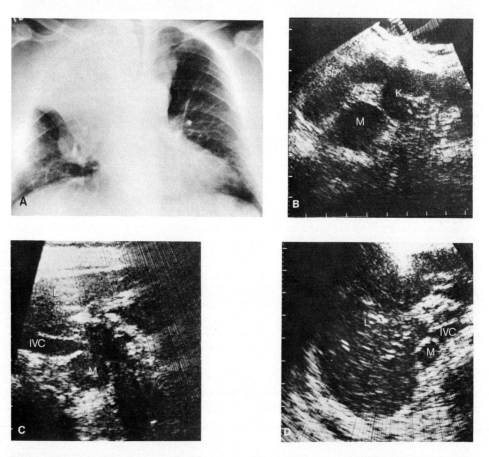

Figure 13. (A) Chest radiograph. An oat cell carcinoma is present and has replaced the right upper lobe. The right hilum is also involved. (B) Sagittal sonogram. A lucent left adrenal mass (M) is seen. (Sp) Spleen; (K) kidney. (C) Sagittal sonogram. A lucent right adrenal mass (M) is seen posterior to the inferior vena cava (IVC). (L) Liver. (D) Transverse sonogram. The relationship between the right adrenal mass (M) and the inferior vena cava (IVC) is again visible and readily explains why the adrenal projects posterior to the IVC on sagittal sections.

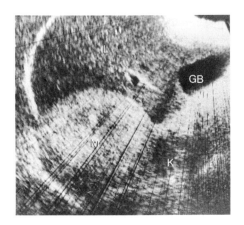

Figure 14. Sagittal sonogram. An echogenic mass (M) has replaced the right adrenal gland. This appearance is compatible with diagnosis of myelolipoma. Note posterior displacement of the diaphragm due to low velocity of sound through fat. The presence of fat was confirmed upon CT. (L) Liver; (K) kidney; (GB) gallbladder.

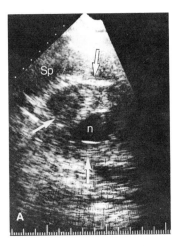

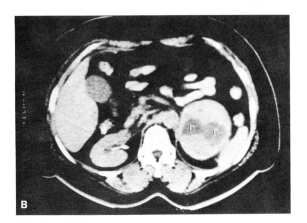

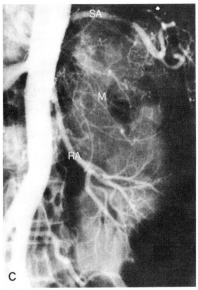

Figure 15. (A) Coronal sonogram. A heterogeneous mass with an area of necrosis (n) has replaced the left adrenal (arrows). (Sp) spleen. (B) CT after intravenous injection of contrast medium. A mass replacing the left adrenal gland is again noted (M). Several areas of necrosis (n) lack contrast enhancement. (C) Aortography. Splaying of the renal artery (RA) and splenic artery (SA) by a vascular mass (M) is visible. A pheochromocytoma was confirmed upon surgery.

The diagnostic approach to an adrenal mass should largely be based on clinical suspicion. If a pheochromocytoma is suspected, CT should be used to evaluate other potential sites of disease (34). These include the para-aortic regions, mediastinum and organ of Zuckerkandl. When a functioning adrenal tumor or hyperplasia is being considered, [^{131}I]iodocholesterol scanning in conjunction with adrenal venous sampling provides the most clinically useful information.

Ultrasound is capable of demonstrating adrenal cysts, hemorrhage, carcinoma, myelolipomas, pheochromocytomas and metastases (Figure 13). Although these tumors are generally solid, they at times can appear quite lucent from hemorrhage or necrosis. Tumors cause the adrenal gland to take on an irregular globular shape. Myelolipomas are tumors consisting of marrow and fatty elements and have a highly echogenic appearance. As with the angiomyolipoma of the kidney, the ultrasound appearance coupled with characteristic fat density on CT is virtually diagnostic (Figure 14) (37).

Pheochromocytomas are variable in their appearance, ranging from homogeneously echogenic to heterogeneous lesions with multiple lucent spaces (Figure 15) (38). On the basis of their sonographic appearance, it is impossible to distinguish benign from malignant lesions. If invasion or metastatic spread can be detected, the lesion can be presumed malignant. Ultrasound as well as CT can be used to follow patients postoperatively for recurrence.

Many potential pitfalls exist in adrenal sonography. It may be difficult to distinguish adrenal lesions from lesions involving the upper pole of the kidney. The spleen, gastroesophageal junction and a tortuous splenic or left renal artery may all mimic a left adrenal mass. The caudate lobe of the liver and second portion of the duodenum may produce confusion on the right (39).

BLADDER

Transabdominal as well as transrectal ultrasound is capable of demonstrating intrinsic and extrinsic neoplastic processes that involve the bladder (40, 42). Little has been published on ultrasound of the bladder. This is partially due

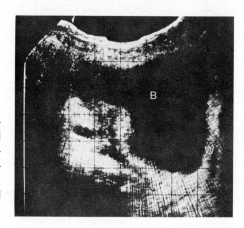

Figure 16. Transverse sonogram. Perivesical tumor spread (T) and bladder wall thickening secondary to this bladder carcinoma can be seen. Note the normal thickness of the contralateral bladder wall (W). (B) Bladder (courtesy of the British Journal of Radiology).

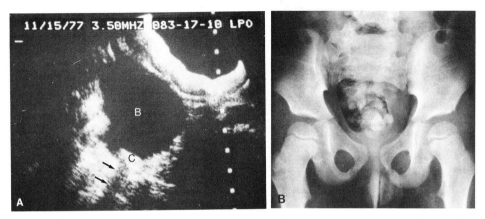

Figure 17. (A) Sagittal sonogram. An echogenic mass with acoustic shadowing (arrows) represents a bladder calculus (C). (B) Bladder. (B) Plain radiograph. Multiple calcified bladder stones were confirmed radiographically.

to the need for cystoscopy and biopsy in many cases and the superiority of CT in assessing side wall extension of pelvic masses. In addition, bladder tumors may produce blood and debris, which makes the bladder wall difficult to define. When performing transabdominal scans, one must examine the bladder in the distended state. The highest frequency transducer, which will allow adequate definition of the perivesical soft tissues, should be used. Transverse and longitudinal sector scans are performed routinely, with decubitus scans being

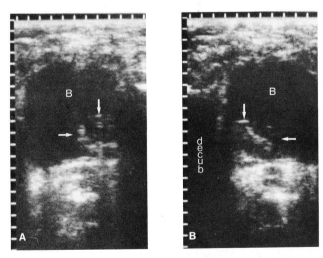

Figure 18. (A) Stopped frames from real-time linear-array scans, transverse sonogram. An echogenic mass (arrows) is resting against the posterior bladder wall. (B) Transverse sonogram. Right lateral decubitus position. The echogenic bladder mass shifted with change in patient position. This is indicative of blood clot. A small transitional tumor was found to be responsible for the patient's hematuria, but this was not seen on sonography.

added to determine whether intravesical contents layer in the dependent position.

The majority of bladder tumors are epithelial in origin and of varying degrees of malignancy. Pedunculated, sessile and intramural infiltrating tumors may be visualized sonographically (40). Invasion of deep tissues may be seen as a local loss of bladder wall definition with echo-poor tumor spreading into the perivesical fat (Figure 16). Lesser degrees of extension may be manifest simply as a local loss of bladder wall distensibility.

Bladder calculi may mimic focal bladder wall abnormalities, especially as they rest against the posterior bladder wall when the patient is in the supine position. Demonstration of acoustic shadowing is seen with larger calculi (Figure 17). Organized clot may appear quite echogenic and also mimic a bladder tumor. Altering patient position will demonstrate movement of the blood clot (Figure 18). Carcinoma of the prostate, uterus and adnexa or bowel may invade the bladder and mimic intrinsic bladder lesions (Figure 19). The location of

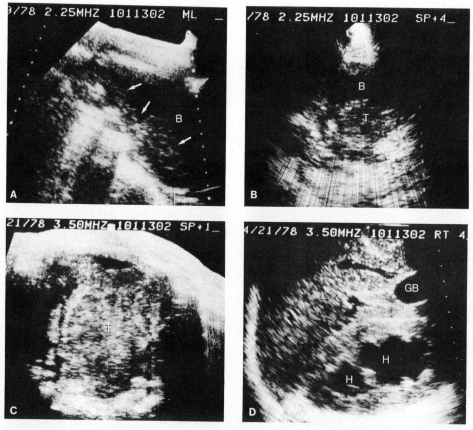

Figure 19. (*A*) Sagittal sonogram. An irregular mass (arrows) is seen protruding into the posterior bladder wall. (B) Bladder. (*B*) Transverse sonogram. This large tumor (T) is seen behind the bladder (B). This appearance suggests prostatic carcinoma invading the bladder. (*C*) Transverse sonogram, 3 months later. The prostatic tumor (T) has increased in size. (*D*) Sagittal sonogram. The tumor has also produced right hydronephrosis (H). (L) Liver; (GB) gallbladder.

the bulk of the mass, the clinical setting and the behavior of the lesion over time will help distinguish these tumors.

REFERENCES

1. Rosenfield AT, Taylor KJW, Crade M, et al: Anatomy and pathology of the kidney by gray-scale ultrasound. Radiology 128: 737–744, 1978.
2. Cook JH, Rosenfield AT, Taylor KJW: Ultrasonic demonstration of intrarenal anatomy. AJR 129: 831–835, 1977.
3. Zeman RK, Cronan JJ, Viscomi GN, et al: Coordinated imaging in the detection and characterization of renal masses. CRC Crit Rev Diag Imaging 15: 273–318, 1981.
4. Pollack HM, Edell SF, Morales JO: Radionuclide imaging in renal pseudotumors. Radiology 111: 639–644, 1974.
5. Bosniak MA: Nephrotomography: A relatively unappreciated but extremely valuable diagnostic tool. Radiology 113: 313–321, 1974.
6. Cronan JJ, Zeman RK, Rosenfield AT: Comparison of computerized tomography, ultrasound, and angiography in the staging of renal cell carcinoma: J Urol 127: 712–714, 1982.
7. Leopold GR, Talner LB, Asher WM, et al: Renal ultrasonography: an updated approach to the diagnosis of the renal cyst. Radiology 109: 671–678, 1973.
8. Rosenfield AT, Taylor KJW: Gray-scale nephrosonography: current status. J Urol 117: 2–6, 1977.
9. Sommer FG, Filly RA, Minton MJ: Acoustic shadowing due to refractive and reflective effects. Am J Roentgenol 132: 973–977, 1979.
10. King DL: Renal ultrasonography—an aid in the clinical evaluation of renal masses. Radiology 105: 633–640, 1972.
11. Green WM, King DL, Casarella WJ: A reappraisal of sonolucent renal masses. Radiology 121: 163–171, 1976.
12. Witten DM, Myers GH, Utz DC: Tumors of the kidney, renal pelvis and ureter. In Emmett's Clinical Urography, 4th Edition. Philadelphia, WB Saunders Co, 1979, pp 1486–1487.
13. Robson CJ, Churchill BM, Anderson W: The results of radical nephrectomy for renal carcinoma. J Urol 101: 297–301, 1969.
14. Skinner DG, Vermillion DC, Colvin RB: The surgical management of renal carcinoma. J Urol 107: 705–710, 1972.
15. Coleman BG, Arger PH, Mulhern CB, et al: Gray-scale sonographic spectrum of hypernephromas. Radiology 137: 757–765, 1980.
16. Maklad MF, Chuang VP, Doust BD, et al: Ultrasonic characterization of solid renal lesions: echographic, angiographic and pathologic correlation. Radiology 123: 733–739, 1977.
17. Green B, Goldstein HM, Weaver RM: Abdominal pan-sonography in the evaluation of renal cancer. Radiology 132: 421–424, 1979.
18. Witten DM, Myers GH, Utz DC: Tumors of the kidney, renal pelvis, and ureter. In Emmett's Clinical Urography, 4th Edition. Philadelphia, WB Saunders Co, 1979, pp 1560–1572.
19. Arger PH, Mulhern CB, Pollack HM, et al: Ultrasonic assessment of renal transitional cell carcinoma: preliminary report. AJR 132: 407–411, 1979.

20. Federle MP, McAninch JW, Kaiser JA, et al: Computed tomography of urinary calculi. AJR 136: 255–258, 1981.

21. Witten DM, Myers GH, Utz DC: Tumors of the kidney, renal pelvis, and ureter. In Emmett's Clinical Urography, 4th Edition. Philadelphia, WB Saunders Co, 1979, pp 1486–1487.

22. Markle BM, Potter BM: Surgical diseases of the urinary tract. In Haller JO, Shkolnik A (eds): Clinics in Diagnostic Ultrasound, Ultrasound in Pediatrics. New York, Churchill-Livingstone, Inc, 1981, pp 135–164.

23. Slovis TL, Phillippart AI, Cushing B, et al: Evaluation of the inferior vena cava by sonography and venography in children with renal and hepatic tumors. Radiology 140: 767–772, 1981.

24. Potter BM, Frank JL: Cancer in the pediatric patient. In Brascho DJ, Shawker TH (eds): Abdominal Ultrasound in the Cancer Patient. New York, John Wiley & Sons, 1980, pp 299–346.

25. Lalli AF: Lymphoma in the urinary tract. Radiology 93: 1051–1054, 1969.

26. Hawn FJY, Peterson NL: Renal lymphoma simulating adult polycystic disease. Radiology 122: 655–656, 1977.

27. Wagle DG, Moore RH, Murphy GP: Secondary carcinomas of the kidney. J Urol 114: 30–32, 1975.

28. Lee TG, Henderson SC, Freeny PC, et al: Ultrasound findings of renal angiomyolipoma. J Clin Ultrasound 6: 150–155, 1978.

29. Hartman DS, Goldman SM, Friedman AC, et al: Angiomyolipoma: Ultrasonic pathologic correlation. Radiology 139: 451–458, 1981.

30. Ambos MA, Bosniak MA, Valensi QJ, et al: Angiographic patterns in renal oncocytomas. Radiology 129: 615–622, 1978.

31. Jander HP: Renal oncocytoma, a nonentity. Radiology 130: 815–817, 1979.

32. Thornbury JR, McCormick TL, Silver TM: Anatomic/radiologic classification of renal cortical nodules. Am J Radiol 134: 1–7, 1980.

33. Sample WF: Adrenal ultrasonography. Radiology 127: 461–466, 1978.

34. Thomas JL, Bernardino ME, Samaan NA, et al: CT of pheochromocytoma. AJR 135: 477–482, 1980.

35. Yeh HC, Mitty HA, Rose J, et al: Ultrasonography of adrenal masses: usual features. Radiology 127: 467–474, 1978.

36. Yeh HC, Mitty HA, Rose J, et al: Ultrasonography of adrenal masses: unusual manifestations. Radiology 127: 475–483, 1978.

37. Behan M, Martin EC, Muecke EC: Myelolipoma of the adrenal: two cases with ultrasound and CT findings. AJR 129: 993–996, 1977.

38. Bowerman RA, Silver TM, Jaffe MH, et al: Sonography of adrenal pheochromocytomas. AJR 137: 1227–1237, 1981.

39. Sample WF, Sarti DA: Computed tomography and gray scale ultrasonography of the adrenal gland: comparative study. Radiology 128: 377–383, 1978.

40. Morley P: The bladder. In Rosenfield AT (ed): Clinics in Diagnostic Ultrasound, Genitourinary Ultrasonography. New York, Churchill-Livingstone, Inc, 1979, pp 149–157.

41. Bree RL, Silver TM: Sonography of bladder and perivesical abnormalities. AJR 136: 1101–1104, 1981.

42. Harada K, Igari D, Tanashi Y, et al: Staging of bladder tumors by means of transrectal ultrasonography. JCU 5: 388–392, 1977.

17

ULTRASONIC DIAGNOSIS OF MALIGNANT TUMORS OF THE PROSTATE

Hiroki Watanabe

Hiroshi Ohe

Equipment for transrectal ultrasonotomography for the examination of the prostate was successfully developed in 1967 (1–4) (Figure 1). The technique allows complete visualization of the prostate, which in horizontal section is seen to lie in front of the rectum bounded by capsular echoes arising from the prostatic capsule and containing internal echoes produced by the prostatic tissue (1, 2) (Figure 2).

Sixty-eight cases of prostatic cancer have been seen in our clinic since the introduction of the method in 1976, and in this chapter we will describe the ultrasonic diagnostic criteria developed on the basis of this experience.

ULTRASONIC DIAGNOSIS OF PROSTATIC CANCER

The diagnostic criteria of prostatic diseases in transrectal ultrasonotomography (3) are summarized in Table 1.

The normal prostatic section is small and shows a triangular or semilunar pattern. The shape of the prostate is always symmetrical. Capsular echoes are thin, continuous and smooth. Internal echoes are distributed regularly with moderate density. Figure 3 shows an ultrasonotomogram of the normal prostate. The slender shape and symmetrical findings are characteristic.

Ultrasonotomograms of the prostate involved with cancer have no definite pattern but show many kinds of deformity, enlargement and an imbalance between the anteroposterior (A-P) diameter and the lateral diameter (Figures 4 and 5). Even in early cases, the prostatic section is asymmetrical and deformed. Capsular echoes are still continuous but are uneven. Internal echoes are irregular but occasionally decrease because of the attenuation of ultrasound by the cancer tissue (Figure 4).

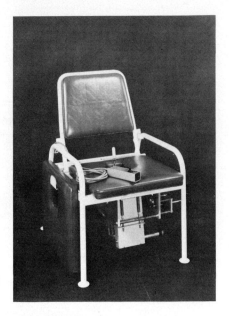

Figure 1.   Special apparatus for transrectal ultrasonotomography.

In advanced cases, deformity and asymmetry are more pronounced. The prostatic section is more enlarged, more commonly affected by A-P diameter elongation, and often shows the so-called bell-shaped pattern (Figure 5A). Elongation of the lateral diameter of the prostate by cancer is rarely seen (Figure 5B). The capsular echoes are irregular and discontinuous. These findings are related to the periprostatic invasion of cancer. Internal echoes are distributed irregularly and somewhat decreased in magnitude.

Another characteristic of a prostate affected by cancer is that horizontal sections at different levels are not analogous (5, 6). The shape of the prostate differs remarkably in the eight sections shown in Figure 6, despite the fact that they were obtained at the same time from one patient.

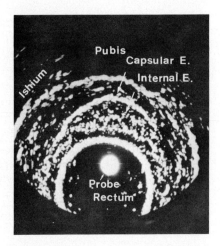

Figure 2.   Horizontal tomogram of the normal prostate.

TABLE 1. Criteria for the Diagnosis of Prostatic Diseases by Transrectal Ultrasonotomography

Findings	Normal	BPH	Prostatic Cancer	Chronic Prostatitis
Shape				
Area	Small	Enlarged	Enlarged in most cases	Usually small
Shape	Triangular or semilunar	Semilunar or circular	Deformed	Somewhat deformed
Symmetry	+	+	−	±
Anteroposterior diameter	Short	Elongated, keeping balance with lateral diameter	Occasionally highly elongated	Short
Capsular echoes				
Thickness	Thin	Thick	Irregular	Irregular
Continuity	+	+	−	−
Evenness	+	+	−	−
Internal echoes				
Quality	Regular	Regular	Irregular	Irregular
Density	Moderate	Increased	Occasionally partially decreased	Occasionally partially decreased
Prostatic shapes on different levels	Analogous	Analogous	Not analogous	Usually analogous

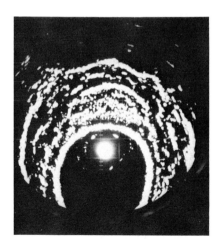

Figure 3. Normal prostate.

233

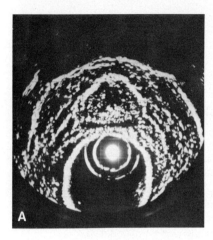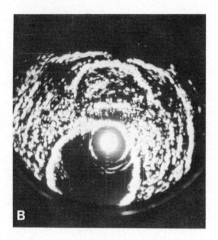

Figure 4.   (*A*) Early prostatic cancer (stage B). The prostate is small but asymmetric. (*B*) Early prostatic cancer (stage B). The deformity is more remarkable than in *A*.

DIFFERENTIAL DIAGNOSIS

Benign Prostatic Hypertrophy (BPH)

The prostatic section in patients with BPH varies from a semilunar shape to a circular shape according to the development of the adenoma. The enlargement is generally symmetrical and there is balance between the A-P diameter and the lateral diameter. The capsular echoes are thick but continuous and smooth. Internal echoes increase and are distributed regularly. These ap-

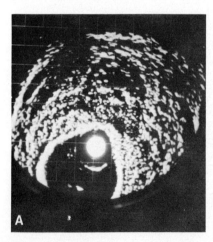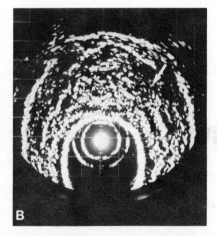

Figure 5.   (*A*) Advanced prostatic cancer (stage C). Remarkable elongation of A-P diameter is observed. (*B*) Advanced prostatic cancer (stage C). Remarkable elongation of the lateral diameter and invasion of the periprostatic tissues can be seen (arrow).

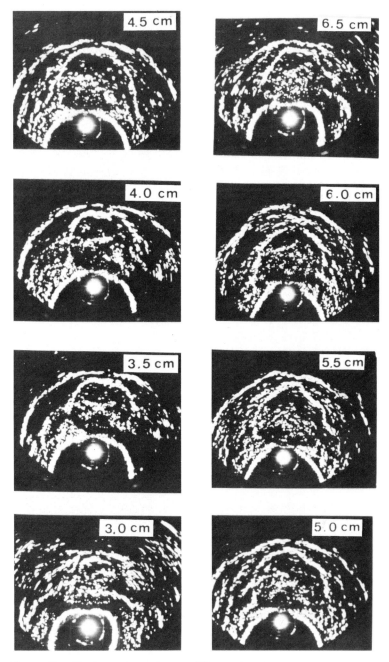

Figure 6. Horizontal section at different levels in prostatic cancer.

235

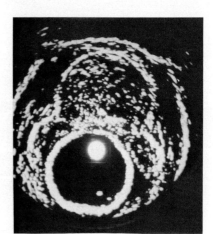

Figure 7.　Horizontal tomogram of BPH.

pearances are quite characteristic and the diagnosis of typical BPH is simple (Figure 7).

Occasionally, advanced BPH coexists with prostatic cancer. In such cases, the differentiation becomes more difficult, as is illustrated by the two cases shown in Figures 8 and 9.

The prostate shown in Figure 8 has a pattern very similar to that of advanced BPH. However, the horizontal sections of the prostate are somewhat asymmetric and not analogous at different levels, suggesting cancer. Needle biopsy of the prostate revealed an adenocarcinoma.

Figure 9 shows an echogram that was interpreted as BPH. Needle biopsy of the prostate supported the interpretation. Subcapsular prostatectomy was performed, and the histological study of the specimen showed several tiny cancer foci. Thus, the diagnosis was prostatic cancer, stage A. Slight asymmetrical distortion of the horizontal section was noticed on careful retrospective evaluation.

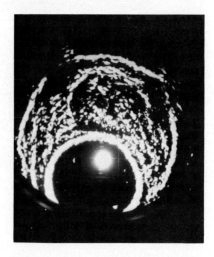

Figure 8.　Prostatic cancer. The image resembles BPH.

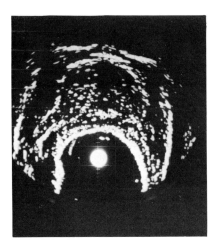

Figure 9. Prostatic cancer, stage A.

Thus, close observation of all sections taken at different levels is necessary to differentiate cancer from BPH. Prostatic shape in BPH is uniform, whereas in cancer it varies.

Chronic Prostatitis

Echograms of chronic prostatitis occasionally resemble those of prostatic cancer (Figure 10), and differentiation sometimes is difficult.

We studied 26 cases of chronic prostatitis in reference to 68 cases of prostatic cancer (7). The contour of the horizontal section of all the cases was traced on the same plan. As shown in Figure 11, the prostate in chronic prostatitis generally is small and somewhat deformed but relatively symmetric in contrast to the prostate in cancer. Capsular echoes often were interrupted, and internal echoes were irregularly distributed.

Symmetry was observed in 85% (22 cases) of the patients with chronic pros-

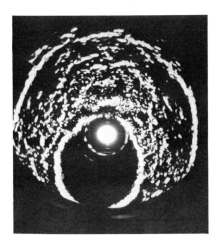

Figure 10. Severe chronic prostatitis.

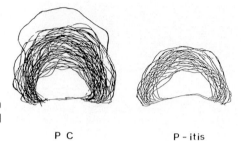

Figure 11. Contour of horizontal section in 68 cases of prostatic cancer (PC) and in 26 cases of chronic prostatitis (P-itis).

P C   P - itis

tatitis but in only 28% (19 cases) of those with prostatic cancer. Prostatic shapes at different levels were analogous in all patients with chronic prostatitis but in only 60% (41 cases) of patients with prostatic cancer.

The prostate in patients with chronic prostatitis was smaller, the estimated average prostatic weight being 19.5 ± 5.5 g in chronic prostatitis compared with 29.4 ± 9.2 g in prostatic cancer.

Thus, the characteristics of chronic prostatitis are a rather small horizontal section symmetrically bounded by an irregular capsule and containing an uneven distribution of internal echoes. These characteristics in many instances allow cancer to be distinguished from infiltration.

ACCURACY OF ULTRASONIC DIAGNOSIS OF PROSTATIC CANCER

To determine the diagnostic accuracy of transrectal ultrasonotomography of prostatic cancer, a survey was made of 3,000 examinations of 2,331 patients with urological diseases (8). This series included the 68 patients with prostatic cancer mentioned above.

Fifty-four (94.7%) of 57 cases diagnosed ultrasonically as prostatic cancer were confirmed by biopsy. Twelve (3.7%) of 326 cases suspected ultrasonically of being prostatic cancer were confirmed by biopsy. Two (0.1%) of 1,741 cases diagnosed ultrasonically as prostatic diseases other than cancer proved to be prostatic cancer. Thus, the false-negative rate in transrectal ultrasonotomography for prostatic cancer was 0.1%. Despite the relatively high false-positive rate, transrectal ultrasonotomography can be considered an excellent screening examination.

STAGING OF PROSTATIC CANCER

The staging of prostatic cancer is very important in determining whether surgery is indicated. According to the American system of classification, stage A includes cancers completely restricted to the prostate and consequently detected incidentally in tissue removed in operations for BPH or on autopsy. Stage B includes cancers that involve almost the whole prostate without ex-

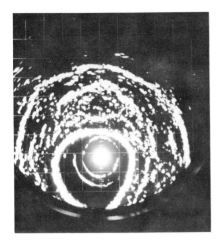

Figure 12. Prostatic cancer, stage B. Capsular echoes are distorted but still continuous.

tracapsular invasion. Stage C refers to cancer invasion beyond the prostatic capsule. Stages A and B indicate surgery.

Whether differentiation between stage A and stage B is possible by the method is still unclear (Figure 9). However, in the stage A cases seen to date, neither deformity nor asymmetry were observed. It is suggested, therefore, that when some deformity is noticed in the section of the prostate the stage should be judged as B. In stage B, the horizontal section of the prostate usually is small, asymmetric and deformed. Capsular echoes are distorted but still continuous (Figures 4 and 12).

Prostatic cancer in stage C is characterized by enlargement, asymmetric and deformed shape, distorted and irregular capsular echoes and partial protrusion of internal echoes beyond the capsular echoes (Figures 5 and 13).

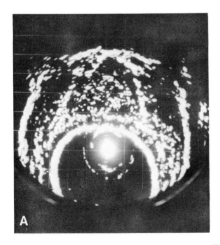
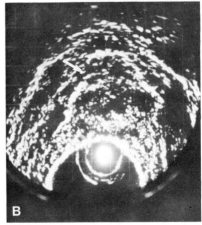

Figure 13. (A) prostatic cancer, stage C. Capsular echoes are interrupted but protrusion of internal echoes beyond the capsule are not remarkable. (B) Prostatic cancer, stage C. Capsular echoes are interrupted, with protrusion of internal echoes (arrow).

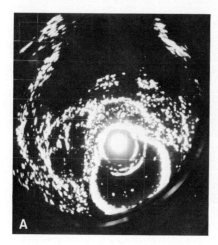 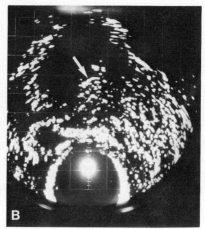

Figure 14. (A) Prostatic cancer, stage D. Echogram shows seminal vesicles dilated and distorted by cancer invasion. (B) Prostatic cancer, stage D. Invasion of bladder neck (arrow).

Igari (9) confirmed that these irregular and discontinuous capsular echoes on ultrasonotomograms coincide with the histological involvement of cancer cells beyond the prostatic capsule.

In some cases, in more advanced stages, infiltrations into the seminal vesicles and bladder neck may be detected ultrasonographically (Figure 14). The seminal vesicles appear dilated and deformed (Figure 15A). A group of irregular fine dots in the bladder neck suggests the intravesical invasion of cancer (Figure 15B). Thus, the location and the degree of cancer invasion can be easily appreciated.

The results of ultrasonic staging were compared with staging by traditional palpation (6). Twenty-nine cases of prostatic cancer were judged as stage B by digital palpation. Cancer infiltration beyond the capsular echoes was detected in 13 of these patients, suggesting that their cancer might be stage C.

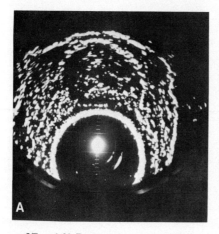 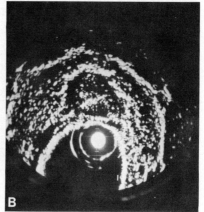

Figure 15. (A) Prostatic cancer before therapy. (B) Prostatic cancer after antiandrogenic therapy.

Total prostatectomy was performed in five patients with prostatic cancer judged as stage B by ultrasound diagnosis. A small periprostatic invasion was detected in one patient by the histological survey of the specimens. Retrospectively, a small interruption of the capsular echoes was noticed in the part where the invasion was pointed out by histology.

EVALUATION OF THE EFFECT OF TREATMENTS FOR PROSTATIC CANCER

The effect of treatment for prostatic cancer can be identified on ultrasonotomograms (3). After hormonal therapy, the shape of the horizontal section of

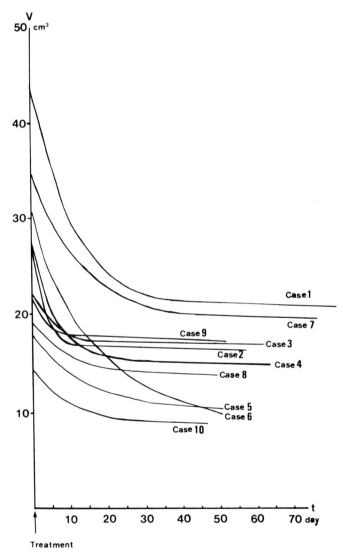

Figure 16.   Regression curve of prostatic volume during treatment for prostatic cancer.

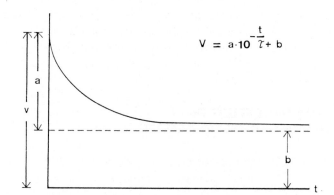

Figure 17. Regression curve and reduction time of the prostate. v = total volume of the prostate; a = effective tissue volume; b = ineffective tissue volume; τ = reduction time.

the prostate is reduced. Capsular echoes become thick and recover continuity. Internal echoes are simplified. These changes usually occur within several weeks from the start of treatment (Figure 15).

It is of practical importance to measure the reduction in volume of the prostate when treating prostatic cancer. Prostatic volume is estimated as the sum of the area of each section taken at 0.5 cm intervals multiplied by 0.5. Studies have shown that the error in this estimation is within 5% (2, 3).

The kinetics of prostatic size reduction during treatment of prostatic cancer has also been analyzed (10). Figure 16 shows the regression curve of prostatic volume estimated by transrectal ultrasonotomography. Prostatic volume decreases exponentially during therapy, approaching a constant plateau level, and this reduction curve may be expressed as $V = a \cdot 10^{-t/\tau} + b$ (Figure 17).

The constant plateau level could indicate the volume of the tissues not af-

TABLE 2.   Effective Portion, Ineffective Portion and Reduction Time

Case	a (cm^3)	b (cm^3)	τ $(days)$
1	24.7	20.8	25.3
2	13.2	16.9	5.8
3	12.0	17.9	6.6
4	7.7	14.5	30.3
5	8.0	9.8	38.7
6	20.4	9.5	37.2
7	15.8	19.5	32.0
8	5.3	14.2	20.9
9	3.6	18.4	3.0
10	5.1	9.2	20.9

fected or responding to the treatment, while the exponentially reduced curve shows the change in the volume of tissues responding to the treatment. Prostatic volume in cancer cases is of course the sum of the effective and the ineffective portions (Figure 17). According to this hypothesis, one can calculate the volume of the effective portion, the ineffective portion and the reduction time, i.e., the time interval required for the effective portion to reduce its volume to one-tenth (Table 2). The figures in Table 2 may represent factors influencing the sensitivity of cancer tissue to the treatment, and investigations are currently underway to further elucidate the relationship between these figures and the prognosis of the patients.

REFERENCES

1. Watanabe H, Kaiho H, Tanaka M, et al: Diagnostic application of ultrasonotomography to the prostate. Invest Urol 8: 548–559, 1971.

2. Watanabe H, Igari D, Tanahashi Y, et al: Development and application of new equipment for transrectal ultrasonotomography. J Clin Ultrasound 2: 91–98, 1974.

3. Watanabe H, Igari D, Tanahashi Y, et al: Transrectal ultrasonotomography. J Urol 114: 734–739, 1976.

4. Watanabe H, Igari D, Tanahashi K, et al: An evaluation of the function of new special equipment for transrectal ultrasonotomography. Tohoku J Exp Med 118: 387–392, 1976.

5. Watanabe H: Prostatic ultrasound. In Rosenfield AT (ed): Genitourinary Ultrasonography. New York, Churchill Livingstone, 1979, pp 125–137.

6. Watanabe H: Prostatic cancer. In Watanabe H, Holmes JH, Holm HH, Goldberg BB (eds): Diagnostic Ultrasound in Nephrology and Urology. Tokyo, Igaku-Shoin Ltd, 1981, pp 130–135.

7. Ohe H, Watanabe H, Saitoh M, et al: Ultrasonotomography of prostatic cancer (1st report)—Reevaluation of diagnostic criteria for prostatic cancer. JSUM Proceedings. 38: 91–92, 1981.

8. Watanabe H, Date S, Ohe H, et al: A survey of 3000 examinations by transrectal ultrasonotomography. The Prostate 1: 271–278, 1981.

9. Igari D: Clinical studies on the prostatic volume and shape by means of transrectal ultrasonotomography. Jpn J Urol 67: 28–39, 1076.

10. Ohe H, Saitoh M, Tanaka S, et al: Kinetics of prostatic size reduction in treating prostatic cancer. JSUM Proceedings 35: 313–314, 1979.

18

ULTRASONIC IMAGING OF TESTICULAR TUMORS

Jack Jellins

Thomas S. Reeve

George Kossoff

Kaye A. Griffiths

Ultrasonic imaging is a noninvasive technique that readily demonstrates the contents of the scrotum. Uniformity of the anatomy enables variations in tissue texture within the testes to be easily recognized, and the technique therefore is able to reveal morphological disturbances in their early stages of development. The technique allows rapid assessment of intratesticular tumors and, in some instances, can indicate before surgical confirmation the morphological nature of the tumor content.

EXAMINATION TECHNIQUE

Examination of the scrotal contents of patients began at the Royal North Shore Hospital in 1975. More than 200 patients have been examined by the open-tank technique of coupling, initially with the Ultrasonics Institute 4-MHz waterbath scanner and more recently with the Ausonics Pty. Ltd. Octoson and System 1. The scrotum is always shaved to minimize artifacts, and the penis is strapped with waterproof adhesive tape to the lower part of the abdomen. Coupling to the patient is best achieved with the patient in a prone position. Both sagittal and coronal planes are scanned in increments of 2 mm. Compound and simple scans are required for the interpretation of the echograms because each mode of scanning provides different textural information. Care must be taken with compound scans to ensure that the degree of compounding is kept to the minimum required to give good images. Both testes are routinely examined to facilitate the recognition of abnormal structures by comparing the area of interest with the normal anatomy.

TABLE 1.   Benign and Malignant Conditions

Benign Conditions	
Fibrosis	18
Epididymitis	18
Epididymo-orchitis	6
Granuloma	2
Lipoma in the spermatic cord	1
Adenomatoid	1
Inguinal hernia	1
	47
Malignant Conditions	
Seminoma	9
Teratoma	3
Embryonal	2
Mixed	2
	16

RESULTS

The echographic appearance of benign and malignant scrotal pathology has been described in a number of publications. In the present series of 200 patients examined by ultrasonography from November 1975 to April 1982, there were 63 with predominantly solid tumors attributed to benign and malignant tissue changes. Of these, 16 were confirmed at biopsy to be malignant. Table 1 shows the types of solid benign and malignant conditions visualized in the clinic.

The most common solid benign changes were associated with inflammatory disease. Eighteen cases of fibrosis were visualized. This condition can be recognized by the isolated areas of increased high-level echoes originating from within the testis. A further 18 cases of epididymitis were visualized. In these patients, the epididymis undergoes changes in both reflectivity and size. Usually there is an increase in the magnitude of the reflected echoes from the epididymis as well as a thickening of the structure.

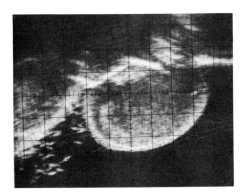

Figure 1. Compound scan of a testis with unusual features within the body of the testis.

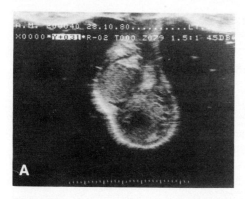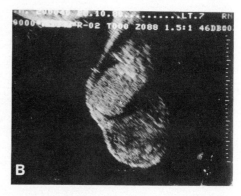

Figure 2. Compound (*A*) and simple (*B*) scans of the scrotal contents. A benign tumor is shown in the left testis. The right testis has a normal appearance.

Intratesticular tumors cause the most concern because it is generally within the body of the testis that malignancies arise. Any change in tissue texture within the body of the testis must be regarded with suspicion, unless the change can be solely attributed to a benign process.

A sagittal compound scan through the body of the testis is shown in Figure 1. The testis is displayed in this plane as an elliptical structure containing echoes of varying levels. In a normal testis the distribution of echoes is more uniform. This image represents a testis that has undergone morphological tissue changes. In the posterior region there is a 1 × 1.5-cm area of low-level echoes with unusual features that suggest a tumor. The body of the testis is circumscribed by the scrotal wall, which normally is displayed with higher-level echoes. Posterior to the testis is the epididymis, containing medium- to high-level echoes. Although there were definite changes noted within the testis, the condition remained unaltered for a number of years and surgery was not thought to be indicated.

Figure 2 shows compound and simple scans of a benign granuloma in the left testis. The tumor disrupts the homogeneous texture of the testis and contains predominantly low- to medium-level echoes. The boundary of the tumor is not clearly demonstrated by either mode of scanning. The simple scan, however, indicates that the texture of most of the testis has been altered.

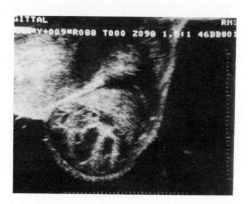

Figure 3. Traumatic disorganization of the testicular tissues.

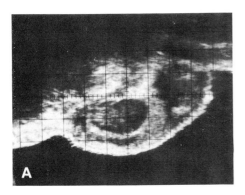 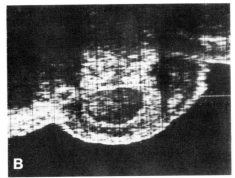

Figure 4.   Images of a well-defined seminoma in the left testis. (*A*) Compound scan. (*B*) Simple scan. The right testis has a normal appearance.

Many changes within the testis are due to damage to the tissues caused by injury or surgical intervention. The testis shown in Figure 3 contains fibrotic septa separated by liquid-filled areas. This gross appearance is restricted to the anterior portion of the testis. The surrounding remaining testicular tissue is homogeneous. A hydrocele is displayed in the superior part of the scrotum.

The presence of malignant tumors extensively modifies the echographic appearance of the testis. A 2 × 3-cm seminoma is shown in the compound scan of the left testis in Figure 4a. The tumor contains echoes that predominantly are low in amplitude, and it is surrounded by a capsule displayed with echoes higher in amplitude than those originating from the testicular tissue. The echoes from within the tumor are lower in amplitude than those from the surrounding testicular tissue but similar in amplitude to the echoes from the other testis. The simple scan shown in Figure 4B better demonstrates the fine detail of the tissue texture.

Not all seminomas produce predominantly low-level echoes. Advanced cases show heterogeneous echoes due to the various tissue structures present. Figure 5 shows a 5 × 4-cm tumor in the right testis. The image is displayed with greater intensity than normal to demonstrate all the detail within the tumor, and, consequently, the contents of the left testis are overwritten.

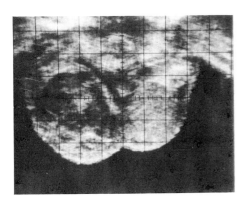

Figure 5.   Echogram of a heterogeneous seminoma in the right testis.

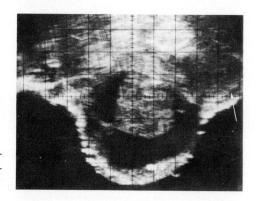

Figure 6. Teratoma with echoes of various levels in the left testis. The right testis is indicated by the arrow.

The teratomas visualized in this series contained echoes of various levels, many of which were stronger than the normal testicular tissue. With the gross structural disorganization present in these tumors, liquid-filled areas of various sizes were always seen. A coronal scan showing a teratoma 4 cm in diameter surrounded by a large hydrocoele is shown in Figure 6. The tumor has replaced the normal tissue and is displayed with both high- and low-level echoes. The scrotal wall is thickened due to the reactive edematous process. The left testis, with a normal distribution of echoes, can be seen in the right-hand part of the echogram.

With larger teratomas, the tissues are even more grossly disrupted Figure 7 shows the echo pattern of an advanced teratoma measuring 6 × 7 cm in cross section. There are numerous areas of high-level echoes from the cartilagenous tissue present as well as echo-free regions representing the liquid-filled cysts.

Two cases of embryonal carcinoma have been visualized. Figure 8 shows an embryonal carcinoma with seminomatous differentiation occupying an area 3 cm in diameter in the left testis of the patient. The echographic appearance is variable throughout the tumor. A similar appearance is demonstrated by an embryonal carcinoma coexisting with a teratoma (Figure 9). The right testis is grossly enlarged, measuring 6 × 9 cm in cross section. The echo pattern in this simple scan is variable and similar to that obtained with the advanced teratoma. The left testis is displayed with a higher intensity in an attempt to demonstrate all the contents of the tumor in the right testis.

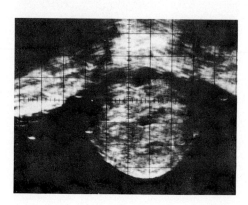

Figure 7. Advanced teratoma with a complex echo pattern.

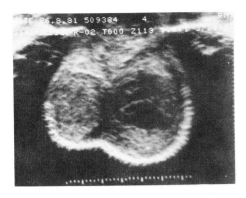

Figure 8. Variable echographic appearance found in an embryonal carcinoma with seminomatous differentiation.

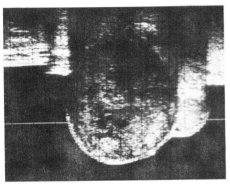

Figure 9. Embryonal carcinoma coexisting with a teratoma.

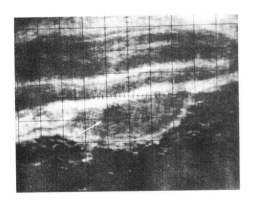

Figure 10. Scan of the right testis showing an area of low-level echoes (the arrow points to the region).

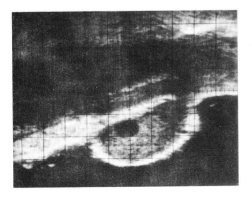

Figure 11. Repeat scan of the right testis with a well-defined tumor, a 12-mm impalpable seminoma.

249

DISCUSSION

Intratesticular tumors can be readily visualized, but the differentiation between benign and malignant changes is difficult. Any change in the tissue texture must be treated with suspicion, but the results of the series described in this chapter indicate that not all variations in texture are due to the presence of a malignancy. In the 200 patients examined, there were 16 cases of confirmed malignancy and a further 14 cases that, although reported as consistent with a malignant change, have not yet been confirmed by surgery. However, any tissue change must be examined thoroughly. The patient whose sonogram is shown in Figure 4 was routinely scanned 18 months after left orchidectomy and radiotherapy treatment. The low-level echo region shown in the posterior part of the right testis in Figure 10 was suggestive of a tissue change but not sufficiently distinct for a definite diagnosis to be made. A further examination, shown in Figure 11, was performed 6 months later. The area visualized previously with echoes slightly lower in amplitude than the surrounding testicular tissue had decreased significantly in echo content. This tumor was impalpable, and biopsy of the area confirmed the presence of a seminoma measuring 12 mm in cross section.

CONCLUSION

Ultrasonic imaging is now an established technique in the visualization of the contents of the testis. It is the method of choice in the preoperative assessment of patients with scrotal enlargements and should be considered mandatory as a routine follow-up procedure in those patients with a history of testicular tumors.

REFERENCES

1. Jellins J, Barraclough BH: Ultrasonic imaging of the scrotum. In White D, Lyons T (eds): Ultrasound in Medicine, Vol 4. New York, Plenum Press, 1978, pp. 151–154.
2. Sample WF, Gottesman JE, Skinner DG, et al: Gray scale ultrasound of the scrotum. Radiology, 127: 225–228, 1978.
3. Leopold GR, Woo VL, Scheible FW, et al: High resolution ultrasonography of scrotal pathology. Radiology, 131: 719–722, 1979.
4. Kossoff G, Jellins J, Reeve TS, et al: Ultrasonic visualisation of scrotal contents. In Watanabe H, Holmes JH, Holm HH, Goldberg BB (eds): Diagnostic Ultrasound in Urology and Nephrology. Tokyo, Igaku Shoin, 1981, pp. 203–210.

19

ULTRASONIC DIAGNOSIS OF GYNECOLOGIC TUMORS

Hisaya Takeuchi

ULTRASONOGRAM OF THE NORMAL FEMALE PELVIS

Vagina

The vaginal canal is visualized as a strong interface on echograms. In longitudinal scans, it is seen as a line that starts at the lower edge of the uterine cervix and runs caudad parallel to the posterior wall of the bladder (Figure 1). In transverse scans, it is seen to be almost parallel to the posterior wall of the bladder, with a width of 1–2 cm. It is surrounded by low-amplitude echoes.

Pelvic Sidewall Musculature

The muscles of the pelvic sidewall and of the pelvis can be imaged if the scan is performed with the transducer tilted at an appropriate angle. In scans performed with the transducer angled at about 10° cephalad, the piriformis muscles can be resolved (Figure 2). Angling 10° caudad reveals the obturator internus muscles. The iliopsoas muscle is seen in the cephalad region. The textural structure of these muscles returns rather low-level echoes, and these must be differentiated from the ovaries.

Vasculature

Although the iliac vessels are quite thick, they are not easily resolved by transverse scanning. They should appear tubelike and run along the vessels, but it is not always easy to determine which vessel is being imaged. It has been suggested (1) that it is easy to identify blood vessels near the ovaries and that longitudinal scans be used to locate the area where the vessels enter the ovary. This procedure is useful for the positive identification of the ovaries (1)

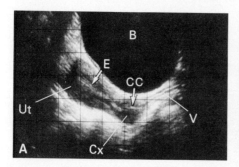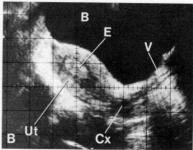

Figure 1. Longitudinal echograms of the normal uterus demonstrating endometrial patterns. (*A*) The linear endometrial pattern. (*B*) The massive endometrial pattern. B, bladder; CC, cervical canal; Cx, cervix; E, endometrium; Ut, uterine body; V, vagina.

(Figure 3). The internal iliac vessels are often seen in contact behind the ovaries.

Ureter

As are the blood vessels, the ureter is in a location that allows it to be imaged, but in practice it is not always easily visualized. The position of the orifice of the ureter can be ascertained by observing in the real-time image the flow of intermittently discharged urine into the bladder.

Uterus

The uterus is secured on both sides by supporting tissue and is connected to the vaginal canal. Thus, it is difficult to displace the cervix from its normal anatomical position. In longitudinal scans, it is generally possible to image the cervix in a section that runs from the umbilicus to the symphysis pubis. In transverse scans the uterine cervix is visualized near the midline in section directly above the symphysis pubis.

The uterus is most clearly demonstrated by a longitudinal scan running along its long axis (Figure 1). The uterine body, fundus and cervix can all be

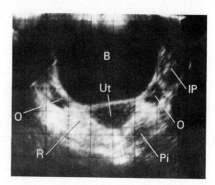

Figure 2. Transverse echogram through both ovaries. B, bladder; IP, iliopsoas muscle; O, ovary; Pi, piriformis muscle; R, rectum; Ut, uterine body.

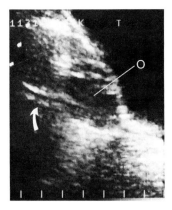

Figure 3. Ovarian vessels (arrow) passing through the infundibulopelvic ligament and entering the ovary are best demonstrated in oblique scans. O, ovary.

demonstrated on a single echogram. When the bladder is filled, the uterus may be slightly off-center, in many cases shifted to the left.

The interval image of the uterus varies with the stages of the menstrual cycle. Immediately after the menstrual phase, the uterine muscles have a weak, grainy echo pattern and the uterine cavity has a relatively weak echo. In mid-menstruation, the period centering around ovulation, the internal echo is linear, a pattern believed to represent the endometrium (Figure 1A). A clumpy endometrial echo and a halo surrounding it are characteristic of the postovulatory phase (Figure 1B). This halo can also be seen in echogram with linear echo.

In childhood the uterine body is smaller than the cervix. The body grows quite markedly during menarche, its width and thickness surpassing that of the cervix. Sample et al (2) have estimated the normal length of the nulliparous uterus in caucasian women to range from 5 to 8 cm and the diameter to range from 1.5 to 3 cm, with means of 6.7 and 2.5 cm, respectively.

Ovary

The situation of the ovaries varies according to such factors as the degree of bladder filling, fullness of the rectum and configuration of the uterus. Nevertheless, its position is limited to behind the bladder, and normal ovaries usually can be delineated (Figure 2). Hackelöer and Nitschke-Dabelstein (1) introduced the method of confirming the ovaries by demonstrating the blood vessels that enter the ovaries (Figure 3). It is difficult to predict the location of the ovaries. They may even be found superior to the uterus or shifted to the opposite side of the uterus.

The shape of the ovary resembles that of a fava bean, and, according to Morley and Barnett (3), measures $1 \times 2 \times 3$–5 cm. Sample et al (2), using a $1/2 \times$ width $\times$ thickness $\times$ length formula, calculated the volume of the ovaries and found them to measure 1.8–5.7 cm^3 in adult women, with a mean of 4.0 cm^3. Cases in which the two diameters exceed 2 cm or the volume exceeds 6.0 cm^3 should be considered abnormal.

The ovaries generally give a low-amplitude diffuse echo pattern, although resolution of small functional cysts is not uncommon.

Bowel

The sigmoid colon and the rectum may be visualized in areas where they are in contact with the uterus. Generally, echoes are obtained only in the anterior wall, accompanied by posterior shadowing. At times, feces that do not contain gas may be mistaken for tumors.

INTERPRETATION OF ECHOGRAMS OF PELVIC MASSES

The application of ultrasonic imaging to the diagnosis of pelvic masses lies in the following areas:

1)   confirmation of presence or absence of a mass,
2)   determination of the organ of origin, the location of the mass and its relationship to other organs and
3)   evaluation of the configuration, size and internal consistency of the mass.

The internal consistency of the tumor refers to the sonographic appearance of the internal nature of the mass, and can be characterized as cystic, solid or complex. Information obtained by this type of imaging is not directly related to the histologic nature of the mass, but rather to its acoustic properties. Criteria for evaluating pelvic masses include (*a*) size and position of the mass, (*b*) internal consistency and (*c*) definition of borders.

Position and Size

Of all the pelvic organs, it is easiest to determine the position of the uterus. It is seen directly behind the filled bladder and its long axis corresponds almost exactly to the midline, although a slight shift to either the left or right is not uncommon. It is convenient to use the cervix as a landmark in locating the uterus.

There are few problems when a mass is clearly revealed inside the uterus, but there is no simple method of determining whether a mass that is adjacent to the uterus is of uterine origin or if it is merely in contact with the uterus. It must be determined by the morphology of the mass and the internal consistency. Pelvic masses other than those of uterine origin very often originate from adnexal organs, particularly from the ovaries. However, consideration must be given to the possibility of masses originating from the intestine, mesentery, omentum and retroperitoneal space. The frequency of bilateral growth is higher for adnexal masses than for other masses.

It must be determined whether masses that occupy the intrapelvic and/or the abdominal cavity are gynecologic or abdominal. The existence of a huge mass makes demonstration of the uterus difficult. The visualization of the intestine below the mass helps to distinguish abdominal or retroperitoneal masses that enlarge caudad from pelvic masses that enlarge cephalad.

Measuring and recording the size of the mass is basic to interpreting the echograms. However, there is no method of accurately recording the size of a mass, which has a complex, three-dimensional shape. The size may yield valuable information about the tumor. For example, it may aid in differentiating a pelvoabdominal multilocular cystic mass from a mucinous cystadenoma of the ovary.

Internal Consistency of Pelvic Masses

The terms cystic, solid and complex are used to describe the internal consistency of a pelvic mass (Figure 4). These terms refer to the macroscopic morphology and are not concerned with the acoustic quality of the mass on the sonogram. The term cystic is not synonymous with the terms echo-free and sonolucent. An echo may be returned from a cystic mass, whereas a solid mass may produce no echo whatsoever.

For a mass to be considered cystic, its internal substance must be in a liquid or liquidlike state and have an echogram with the following three character-

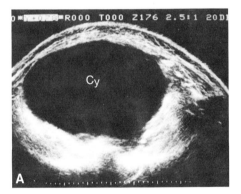

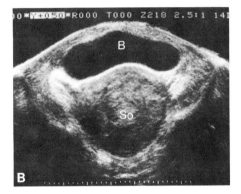

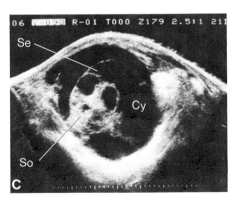

Figure 4. Types of internal consistency of pelvic masses. (A) Cystic mass. This is a typical serous cyst, so its internal consistency is totally echo free. The cyst wall is too thin to be demonstrated. The echo enhancement of the posterior wall is clear. (B) Solid mass. The mildly to moderately echogenic solid mass is a uterine leiomyoma. The boundary is comparatively clear. (C) Complex mass. A moderately echogenic mass is seen within a multilocular cyst with septa. Acoustic shadows do not appear in the solid part. This is a transverse echogram of metastatic ovarian cancer. B, bladder; Cy, cyst; Se, septum; So, solid mass.

istics:

1) well-defined boundries and/or clear wall echo,
2) echo-free or very mildly echogenic contents and
3) echo enhancement of the posterior wall due to good sound transmission (less attenuation).

The presence or absence of septa determines whether the mass is simple or multilocular, and the number of cysts determines whether it is termed single or multiple.

Differences in the echogenicity of solid tumors are due to their histologic and acoustic properties. The border may or may not be well defined. Although a solid tumor with less echo may appear to be cystic at first glance, posterior echo enhancement cannot be observed because of high attenuation.

A technique has been proposed (4) for determining the histology of echogenic masses on the basis of the echo distribution pattern. It must be appreciated that internal echoes can be obtained from a predominantly liquid lesion. For instance, sebaceous material of dermoid cysts, organized clots and purulent debris can give rise to relatively strong internal echoes and appear on the echogram to be of solid texture.

In the case of complex masses, the predominance of either the cystic region or solid region is first determined. Then, attention should be focused on the echogenicity and homogeneity of the solid region. In cystic degeneration of solid masses, the solid region is often homogeneous. Masses whose solid region is largely heterogeneous are often malignant tumors.

Border

The border of a mass is sometimes difficult to demonstrate echographically, particularly when the border of the mass is adjacent to the abdominal wall, intestine or retroperitoneum. Generally no problem is encountered if the mass is surrounded by ascites. Masses with irregular walls usually are malignant, but this irregularity is also seen in inflammatory growth. The internal wall of a cystic mass is easily observed. Differentiation or thickening of the wall itself and layering of debris along the wall are important diagnostic signs.

General Comments

Because ultrasonography does not reveal information about the histology of tissues, it cannot provide the definitive clinical diagnosis. However, in over 90% of masses limited to the pelvis it will provide information concerning the size and internal consistency of the mass.

It goes without saying that the examination would be of great clinical value if it could be used to distinguish benign and malignant tumors. Unfortunately, although malignancy often may be suspected from ultrasonographic results, a definitive histologic diagnosis cannot be made.

Fleischer et al (5) reported a false-positive and false-negative diagnosis rate of 5% in the determination of the presence of tumors. Most of the false-negative results were obtained when the mass lay behind the intestine. Indeed, most misreadings of the scan were due to some factor involving the intestines. When the intestine contains fluid, it is particularly easy to misread the echogram. It is also possible that a urologic organ such as the kidney, ureter or bladder may be mistaken for a pelvic mass.

ULTRASONIC EVALUATION OF UTERINE TUMORS

Uterine tumors that may be detected by ultrasonography include uterine myoma, adenomyosis, sarcoma and endometrial cancer. It is necessary to differentiate such lesions as pyometra, hematometra and bicornuate uterus.

Uterine Myoma (Leiomyoma)

Myoma would be simple to diagnose if the nodule could be clearly demonstrated. However, various types of nodule, ranging from echo-free to markedly echogenic, are seen. The various echogenic properties are due to factors such as the relative proportions of fibrous and muscle tissue in the nodule, secondary changes, such as calcification and hyaline degeneration, and condition of the surrounding uterine muscle layer.

In the usual case, the echo from the nodule is weaker than that from normal muscles, and the border of the nodule is slightly unclear (Figure 5A). The existence of myoma is often predicted on the basis of the irregularity and swelling of the uterine body rather than the delineation of a nodule. The position of the nodule may be predicted on the basis of a shift of the endometrial echo. In cases in which the leiomyoma is more echogenic than normal muscle, the echo enhancement of the tumor's posterior wall can be observed. This is seen when there is an abundant supply of blood, such as during pregnancy or when there is a large amount of muscle tissue.

Increased echogenicity and cystic formation are seen in cases of hyaline degeneration, and it is not uncommon that such cases are misdiagnosed as ovarian masses and even malignant tumors.

Acoustic shadows may also accompany abundant fibrous tissue or marked calcification.

During pregnancy, the echogenicity of a leiomyoma increases, and it becomes easier to visualize the nodule (Figure 6). Often the echogenicity and shape of the nodule change as the pregnancy progresses. Due to the expansion of the uterus, the position of the nodule may also change, sometimes quite dramatically.

The differentiation of pedunculated nodules and solid masses outside the uterus is not easy. Efforts to visualize the peduncle have not always met with success. Bezjian and Carretero (6) advocate applying gentle pressure while scanning as a useful way of determining the relationship of the mass to the

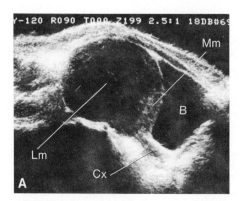

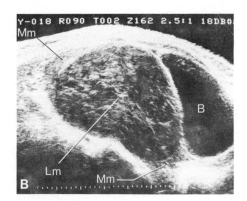

Figure 5. Leiomyoma of the uterus displays many types of echo patterns ranging from essentially echo free to markedly echogenic. (*A*) Markedly reduced echogenicity compared with the normal myometrium. An enlarged mass is seen in the uterine body. (*B*) Almost the same echogenicity as normal myometrium. The acoustic texture within the nodule is extremely homogeneous. (*C*) In a transverse scan, the internal consistency of giant masses that fill the peritoneal cavity can be easily separated into a moderately echogenic solid part and a cystic degeneration caused by leiomyoma. Ao, Aorta; B, bladder; Cy, cyst; Cx, cervix; Lm, leiomyoma; Mm, myometrium.

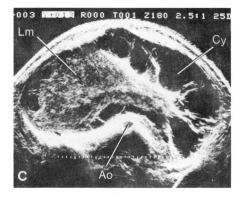

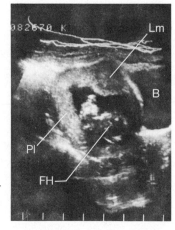

Figure 6. Myoma in the uterine wall at 12 weeks gestation. B, bladder; FH, fetal head; Lm, leiomyoma; Pl, placenta.

258

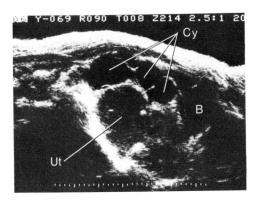

Figure 7. In this longitudinal scan the uterus is enlarged but no nodule is seen and the echogenicity is decreased. Adenomyosis is widespread. In the anterior wall of the uterus what appears to be multiple cysts is seen, but this is really endometrium. B, bladder; Cy, cyst; Ut, uterine body.

uterus. Consideration should be given to the possibility of a bicornuate uterus if a solid mass outside the uterus is observed.

Adenomyosis

Macroscopic observation of the uterus with adenomyosis will not clearly reveal the border between the adenomyosis and normal muscles. This is also true of echographic visualization, which reveals a heterogeneous, rather echo-free texture (Figure 7). Adenomyosis should be suspected if the uterus is enlarged and has a smooth configuration, and particularly if nodules are not observed. A dispersed, coarsely granular echo, the so-called "Swiss cheese" appearance, may be seen within the uterus, when hemorrhage with clots occurs inside the myometrium.

Malignant Uterine Tumors

Swelling of the cervix is seen in advanced cancer of the uterine cervix. There is no unique echo pattern, and diagnosis cannot be made on the basis of the cervical swelling alone. Scanning, therefore, should not be directed at the early diagnosis of the malignancy, but rather at determining the extent of invasion

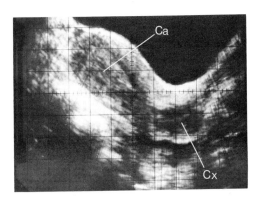

Figure 8. Longitudinal scan of endometrial carcinoma. In the posterior aspect of the uterine body a mildly echogenic mass surrounded by an echo-free halo is seen. Ca, endometrial cancer; Cx, cervix.

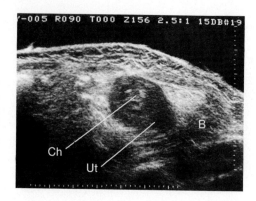

Figure 9. Echogram of choriocarcinoma (Ch). Because of insufficient bladder filling, a longitudinal scan of the uterus reveals only the upper portion of the uterine body (Ut). A cystic region near the fundus of the uterus and an area of increased echogenicity can be seen. B, bladder.

of the adjacent tissue in advanced cases. Transrectal radial scanning has been attempted for this purpose. As yet the ultrasonographic characteristics are not fully understood and problems remain in the interpretation of the echograms.

Since the endometrium can be visualized during the secretory phase, better results may be expected in endometrial cancer (Figure 8). In practice, these expectations are not always realized. Niwa et al (7), using a tumorous endometrial echogram as a criterion for suspecting endometrial cancer, found 8 of 24 cases of clinically suspected cancer. All eight cases were in fact carcinoma, but the false-positive rate was 25% (4 of 16 cases) and the false-negative rate 29.4% (5 of 17 cases). Porranth (8) also reported finding an increased echo in echograms of 6 of 11 cases of endometrial cancer. He also found three normal echograms, four decreased endometrial echoes and one echogram showing both increase and decrease of endometrial echo. It is unlikely, therefore, that abnormal endometrial echoes or tumorous echograms will be obtained in all cases of carcinoma of the uterine body. Intrauterine radial scanning has been performed in an attempt to access the degree of invasion of the cancer to the wall of the uterus (9).

Although choriocarcinoma, like cancer of the uterine body, presents no characteristic echogram, Aoki et al (10) observed an increased echo within the uterine muscles, an echo-free space and tumor echo (clumpy, strong or granular echo with an echo-free space) at the site of lesions. Fleischer et al (11) reported echograms with dense echoes accompanying cystic regions to be characteristic of the necrotic and hemorrhagic part of a tumor. Ultrasonography is useful in the determination of the location of choriocarcinomas (Figure 9).

Several authors (8, 12, 13) are of the opinion that there is no distinctive echogram in uterine sarcoma. It is difficult to differentiate myoma with or without degeneration to sarcoma.

ULTRASONIC EVALUATION OF OVARIAN MASSES

Nontumorous cysts often form in the ovaries, and it is almost impossible to differentiate these functional cysts from cystoma. Echogenicity within the tumor does not necessarily reveal a histologically solid mass, and therefore, the following points should be kept in mind when interpreting echograms of ovarian masses.

Ultrasonography of ovarian masses aims to (*a*) confirm the existence of the mass and (*b*) to reveal its size and internal consistency, which in turn may be expected to assist in determining its type. Below is a classification of ovarian masses based on ultrasonographic pattern.

Cystic: follicle cyst, corpus luteum cyst, lutein cyst, parovarian cyst, endometrioma, serous cystadenoma, polycystic ovary, inflammatory cyst.

Complex: dermoid cyst, mucinous cystadenoma, cystadenocarcinoma, metastatic ovarian cancer.

Solid: dermoid cyst, fibroma, Brenner tumor, solid teratoma, granulosa cell tumor, arrhenoblastoma, dysgerminoma, choriocarcinoma, papillary adenocarcinoma.

Note that there are many nonneoplastic masses in the cystic category and that all malignant masses have a solid part that with proper scanning will be revealed on the echograms.

Nonneoplastic Masses of the Ovary

Follicles

Kratochwil et al (14) reported the demonstration of follicles in normal ovaries, and Hackelöer and Robinson (15) estimated the size of the follicle and were able to monitor its growth. Since then, there have been many reports on the observation of follicle development by ultrasonography.

Follicles with a diameter of more than 1 cm can be identified with certainty (Figure 10). Although several follicles start to develop stimultaneously in both ovaries, only one follicle will enlarge to approximately 2 cm and be ovulated. Follicles grow at a rate of 0.2–0.4 cm a day. Kerin et al (16) reported that nonovulated follicles did not exceed 1.5 cm in diameter. Immediately before reaching its maximum size, the Graafian follicle reveals within it a small mass believed to be the corpus luteum.

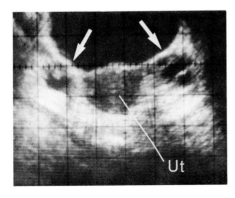

Figure 10. Transverse scan. Cystic regions (arrows) are seen on both sides of the uterus (Ut). These are follicles within the ovaries. One of these has developed to become a Graafian follicle.

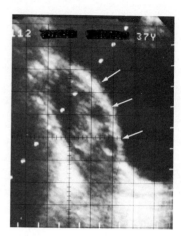

Figure 11. In this longitudinal scan of an enlarged ovary, follicles measuring 1 cm in diameter are seen directly below the ovarian surface (arrows). This is a case of polycystic ovary without Stein-Leventhal syndrome.

Polycystic Ovary

Polycystic ovaries are characterized by numbers of cysts of normal size. There are two types. One type accompanies Stein-Leventhal syndrome. Both ovaries become enlarged, but because the follicles are often less than 5 mm in diameter, they may be too small to be demonstrated on the echogram. Polycystic ovary without Stein-Leventhal syndrome usually is unilateral. The ovary contains a few relatively large follicles (Figure 11).

Hyperstimulation Syndrome

The hyperdevelopment of follicles in cases of hyperstimulation syndrome brought about by induction of ovulation may be clearly revealed by ultrasonography. It can usually be anticipated before hyperstimulation appears. Not only follicles but also stromata become swollen due to edema and are demonstrated as complex masses (Figure 12).

Functional Cysts

Follicles that enlarge but are not ovulated normally are unilocular with thin walls. They rarely grow to be larger than 10 cm. These cysts are difficult to differentiate from serous cystadenoma and other simple cysts.

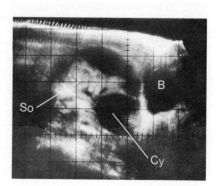

Figure 12. Ovary in a case of hyperstimulation syndrome containing extremely enlarged follicles and hypertrophic parenchyma with edema. B, bladder; Cy, enlarged follicle; So, hypertrophic parenchyma with edema.

Corpus luteum cysts are unilateral simple cysts. They often develop in early pregnancy and may have an echogenic part within the cyst that is due to hemorrhage. Thecal lutein cysts associated with hydatidiform mole and choriocarcinoma are bilateral and multilocular.

Endometriosis

Ovarian endometriosis does not have a characteristic echogram. The mass is not extremely large. Rather than appearing multilocular, it looks more like multiple cysts (Figure 7), and it is not uncommon for it to be bilateral. It may be found in posterior and posterolateral areas of the uterus and often has thick walls. Because of bleeding, weak and diffuse echoes may be observed inside the cyst. Hemosiderin sediment or blood clots may resemble solid parts on the echograms (Figure 13).

Parovarian Cysts

Cysts known as hydatids of Morgagni develop from the Gartner duct. It is not possible to differentiate them from ovarian cysts. They have thin walls, are unilocular and grow to be quite large.

Ovarian Tumors

Histologic diagnosis of ovarian tumors cannot be made by ultrasound. Histologically different tumors often present similar echograms. Nevertheless, a particular type of tumor may have a characteristic sonographic appearance.

Echograms Suggesting Malignant Ovarian Tumors

All malignant tumors of the ovaries have solid malignant tissue. The key to detecting malignant tumors is the interpretation of the areas that appear solid on the echograms, which may be of either the solid or complex type.

The main features of the complex-type echogram are an irregular solid part projecting from the wall into the cavity, loss of definition of the tumor's border

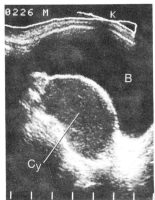

Figure 13. Because the internal consistency of endometrioma is hemorrhagic, a mildly echogenic pattern is not rare. The cyst wall is relatively thick and often clearly revealed. Echo enhancement is not seen in the posterior aspect. B, bladder; Cy, chocolate cyst.

and hypertrophy and projection of the septum. The solid part of the wall or septum that faces the cavity may be irregular and appear acoustically soft.

Solid-type echograms often represent malignant tumors with a characteristic shape such as malignant solid teratoma, dysgerminoma, arrhenoblastoma or papillary adenocarcinoma. The echograms are acoustically soft or hyperechoic, and often display irregularity of echo amplitude. Ascites is often seen in cases of malignant tumor but may also be seen in benign cases as well.

Several Japanese workers, including the author (4, 17), have reported the results of ultrasonic diagnosis of malignant ovarian tumors. Diagnostic criteria were those used for the determination of malignant tumors already described and gave a diagnostic accuracy ranging from 74.1 to 77.4).

Serous Cystadenoma

The size of these tumors varies, but they may grow so large as to occupy part of the abdomen (Figure 14A). The wall is thin and a septum often forms. Bilateral tumors are not uncommon, but determining whether a tumor is bilateral or not is difficult due to the variability of tumor size. Ascites is rarely seen. Differentiation from serous adenocarcinoma with a small solid area is necessary.

Mucinous Cystadenoma

These tumors often are extremely large. They are clearly polycystic with septa of varying thickness (Figure 14B). Thick septa that appear solid suggest malignancy. Mucinous cystadenoma are unilateral and accompanied by less ascites.

Cystadenocarcinoma

Serous and mucinous cystadenocarcinomas are morphologically quite different. Serous cystadenocarcinoma presents a complex-type echogram and has a solid part that protrudes into the cavity (Figure 14C). Diagnosis of malignancy in cases of mucinous cystadenocarcinoma is difficult because there is no great difference between the appearances of the solid part of the malignant tumor and the solid part of benign cystadenoma. In such cases, the loss of definition of the wall provides valuable information.

Metastatic ovarian tumor, known as Krukenberg tumor, is a complex tumor containing abundant solid parts (Figure 14D) and is bilateral.

Pseudomyxoma Peritonei

The peritoneal cavity is filled with mucinous substance, but in contrast to ascites, this substance may take the shape of a mass (Figure 15). The mucinous substance gives a weak echo, which may be sustained.

Dermoid Cyst

Dermoid cysts account for about 25% of all ovarian tumors. They can present a cystic, solid or complex echogram (Figure 16). The cysts are relatively small

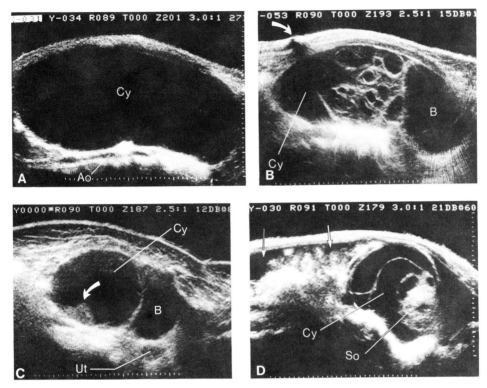

Figure 14. The internal consistency of cystadenoma is either cystic or complex. Care must be taken not to overlook the possible small solid parts. On either side, echo enhancement is clear in the posterior aspect. (*A*) Longitudinal scan of serous cystadenoma. It is an extremely large cyst, but the septum cannot be seen in this scan. (*B*) Many septa are characteristic of mucinous cystadenoma. The septa may appear thick and solid, but careful observation reveals that they differ from malignant solid parts. In this echogram, acoustic shadows are seen in the umbilical region (arrow). (*C*) Primary serous cystadenocarcinoma of the ovary with a small solid part (arrow) in the posterior aspect. Notice the soft, protruded impression the solid part gives. (*D*) This complex-type mass, in which a markedly echogenic solid part is seen, is a Kruckenberg tumor. In general, Krukenberg tumors have a large solid part component. This tumor is accompanied by ascites (arrows). Ao, aorta; B, bladder; Cy, cyst; So, solid part; Ut, uterus.

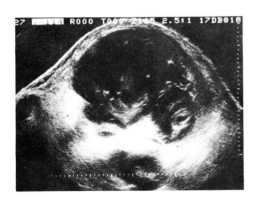

Figure 15. Pseudomyxoma peritonei reveals a variety of patterns. Certain cases have echograms which are similar to those of mucinous cystadenoma, but this case does not reveal a tumorlike structure. The peritoneal cavity appears cystic, but the border is unclear and the picture differs from an echogram showing ascites.

265

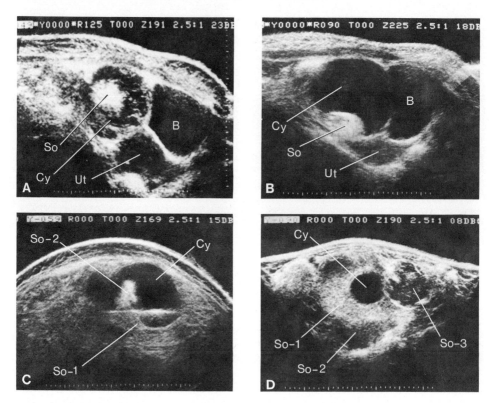

Figure 16. Dermoid cysts demonstrate a variety of appearances. Four patterns are shown here. (*A*) Type in which a solid mass is found within a cystic mass. In this case, the cyst wall is thick and irregular, and the mass contains echoes. The solid mass is markedly echogenic and its borders are irregular. (*B*) Type in which a clear solid part is formed by enlargement of the inside wall of a cystic mass. The texture of the surface of the solid part opposite is smooth, and a dermoid corn may be revealed. (*C*) Type in which the internal consistency can be divided into two parts: anechoic and echogenic. Fluid keeps them separated. Because the cyst contains sebaceous material, this fluid can move easily with the cyst and remains intact even if its position is changed. In this case, the border of the cyst gives rise to an extremely strong linear echo. Echoes from the cartilage (So) are also seen. (*D*) Type in which many moderately echogenic internal components containing cystic parts are found. In the case shown here, very complex components are seen. Moderately echogenic parts (So-1) and mildly echogenic parts (So-2) both have homogeneous echo patterns, which are often encountered in dermoid cysts. There is also a solid part (So-3) and cystic part, which makes a total of four different types of acoustic pattern. B, bladder; Cy, cystic part; So, solid part; Ut, uterine body.

and have thin walls. The borders of solid-type dermoid cysts are indistinct and difficult to identify. In the cystic-type cysts, a dermoid cone may be observed along a portion of the wall. Sebaceous material is easily moved and may form a fluid level with other material. Dental elements may cast an acoustic shadow. Dermoid cysts, while often portrayed by a distinctive echo pattern, may be difficult to differentiate from malignant tumors in cases in which the echogenicity of the solid part is high.

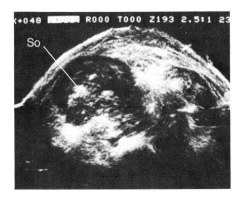

Figure 17. Benign solid teratoma (So). The boundary is indistinct and internal echogenicity markedly heterogeneous. Within the tumor there is little attenuation. So, dermoid corn.

Solid Teratoma

These tumors are often seen in childhood and adolescence and are usually unilateral. Generally, the internal echo pattern is heterogeneous (Figure 17). The tumors may be benign, but clinically must be considered malignant.

Dysgerminoma

Dysgerminomas usually show solid echograms with less irregularity (Figure 18). They are seen often in younger women but are detected only after growing to be quite large. They should be considered clinically malignant.

Granulosa Cell Tumor

Granulosa cell tumors are solid. Because they return homogeneous echoes, they may be difficult to distinguish from uterine myoma. They differ from dysgerminoma in that they are usually seen around menopause.

Arrhenoblastoma (Sertoli-Leydig Cell Tumor)

These are solid tumors whose internal echo patterns are full of irregularity. The echogram cannot be distinguished from echograms of dysgerminoma and granulosa cell tumor. They are rare and should be considered malignant.

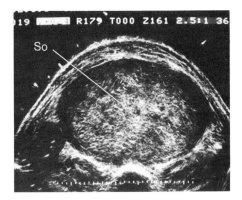

Figure 18. In dysgerminoma, the internal echogenicity is less heterogeneous. Typically, a halo is seen around the boundary. So, dysgerminoma.

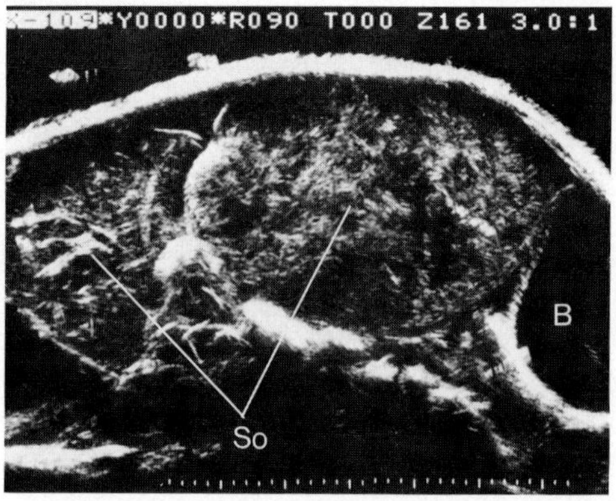

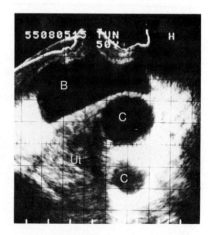

Figure 19.   Generally, ovarian fibroma is mildly echogenic but may be almost totally anechoic. The fibroma in this case is necrotic, causing the echogenicity to increase heterogeneously. B, bladder; So, necrotized ovarian fibroma.

Fibroma

Ovarian fibromas acoustically resemble uterine myoma, although as shown in Figure 19, they tend to have weaker homogeneous echoes. It is difficult to differentiate the two and nearly impossible to differentiate fibroma with degeneration from malignant solid tumor. When associated with ascites and hydrothorax, it is known clinically as Meigs syndrome.

Other Ovarian Tumors

Brenner tumors are solid tumors. Interpretation of scans is difficult when the tumor is in association with mucinous cystadenoma. It is not possible to detect endometrial sinus tumors in association with dermoid cyst. Endometrioid tumor and clear cell tumor do not give rise to characteristic echograms.

Tumors of the Fallopian Tube

Tumors of the fallopian tubes are extremely rare. It is nearly impossible to differentiate them from ovarian and uterine tumors by their location and morphology.

Figure 20.   In hydrosalpinx and pyosalpinx, the fallopian tube expands, and depending upon the angle of the scan, a variety of cysts may be revealed. In this case, the scan cuts the tube in two locations. B, bladder; Cy, hydrosalpinx; Ut, uterine body.

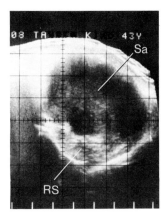

Figure 21. Retroperitoneal tumors are diagnosed echographically by the location of the tumor. In this case, a liposarcoma has forced the blood vessels and lumbar muscles posteriorly. Sarcoma is, in general, an acoustically homogeneous tumor, whereas a liposarcoma essentially is structureless. RS, normal retroperitoneal structures; Sa, liposarcoma.

Differentiation of hydrosalpinx and pyosalpinx from ovarian cyst presents a problem, though by the morphology it is sometimes possible to assume inflammatory disorder of the fallopian tubes (Figure 20).

Retroperitoneal Tumors

Ultrasonography can be used to examine retroperitoneal tumors mistaken for gynecologic tumors. It is often difficult to prove that large tumors are of retroperitoneal origin. With smaller tumors this can be determined by the location of the tumors. Urologic tumors, hematoma, lymphatic cysts, liposarcoma and uterine myoma nodules that enlarge toward the retroperitoneal space are all suited to ultrasonic examination, although other findings also should be considered (Figure 21).

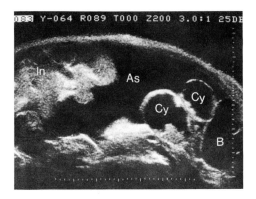

Figure 22. Because the ascites has no boundary and the echo-free part spreads to inside the abdominal cavity, it is not difficult to distinguish it from cystic tumor. During an examination with the patient in the supine position, attention is required since ascites accumulates on both sides of the abdominal region and in the cul-de-sac. When the patient is in the prone position, the ascites collects directly below the abdominal wall. Here a case of metastatic ovarian cancer observed with the patient in the prone position is accompanied by ascites. As, ascites; B, bladder; Cy, metastatic ovarian cancer; In, intestine.

Ascites

Ascites is an important finding in malignant ovarian tumors. The presence or absence of ascites should always be determined in cases in which a malignant ovarian tumor is suspected (Figure 22). An additional scan running from the lateral abdomen to the upper abdomen should be taken with the patient in a supine position. Malignant ovarian tumors can usually be ruled out if ascites is seen to collect in a cul-de-sac, because in malignancy the cul-de-sac is closed off. Although malignant ovarian tumor accompanied by ascites may be suspected, it does not mean that it is peritonitis carcinomatosa.

REFERENCES

1. Hackelöer BJ, Nitschke-Dabelstein S: Ovarian imaging by ultrasound: an attempt to define a reference plane. J Clin Ultrasound 8: 497–500, 1980.
2. Sample WF, Lippe BM, Gyepes M: Gray-scale ultrasonography of the normal female pelvis. Radiology 125: 477–483, 1977.
3. Morley P, Barnett E: The ovarian mass. In Sanders RC, James Jr AE (eds): The Principles and Practice of Ultrasonography in Obstetrics and Gynecology, 2nd ed. New York, Appleton-Century-Crofts, 1980, pp. 357–386.
4. Takeuchi H, Kawamata C, Sugie T, et al: Grey scale ultrasonic diagnosis of ovarian carcinoma. In Kurjak A (ed): Recent Advances in Ultrasound Diagnosis (ICS 436). Amsterdam, Excepta Medica, 1978, pp. 113–121.
5. Fleischer AC, James Jr AE, Millis JB, et al: Differential diagnosis of pelvic masses by gray scale sonography. Am J Roentgenol 131: 469–474, 1978.
6. Bezjian A, Carretero M: Ultrasonic evaluation of pelvic masses in pregnancy. Clin Obstet Gynecol 20: 325–339, 1977.
7. Niwa K, Obata A, Fukumoto S, et al: Studies on the ultrasound tomogram of endometrial cancer. Proceedings of the 33rd Meeting of the Japan Society of Ultrasonics in Medicine, 1978, pp. 175–176.
8. Porrath SA: Ultrasonic evaluation of malignant uterine tumors. In Sanders RC, James Jr AE (eds): The Principles and Practice of Ultrasonography in Obstetrics and Gynecology, 2nd ed. New York, Appleton-Century-Crofts, 1980, pp. 407–425.
9. Sekiba K, Obata A, Akamatsu N, et al: Ultrasound estimation of myometrial invasion of endometrial carcinoma by using intrauterine radial scanning. In Levi S (ed): Ultrasound and Cancer, Amsterdam-Oxford-Princeton, Excerpta Medica, 1982, pp. 147–155.
10. Aoki M, Chiba T, Kanzaki T, et al: Ultrasonographic diagnosis of chorionic tumors. Proceedings of the 34th Meeting of the Japan Society of Ultrasonics in Medicine, 1978, pp. 337–338.
11. Fleischer AC, James, Jr AE, Krause D, et al: Sonographic patterns in trophoblastic disease. Radiology 126: 215–220, 1978.
12. Cochrane WJ: Ultrasound in gynecology. Radiol Clin North Am 13: 457–466, 1975.
13. Lawson TL, Albarelli JN: Diagnosis of gynecologic pelvic masses by gray scale ultrasonography: Analysis of specificity and accuracy. Am J Roentgenol 128: 1003–1006, 1977.

14. Kratochwil A, Urban G, Friedrichs F: Ultrasonic tomography of the ovaries. Ann Chir Gynaecol Fenn 61: 211–214, 1972.

15. Hackelöer BJ, Robinson HP: Ultraschalldarstellung des wachsenden Follikels und Corpus luteum in normalen physiologischen Zyklus. Geburtsh u Frauenheilk 38: 163–168, 1978.

16. Kerin JF, Edmonds DK, Warnes GM, et al: Morphological and functional relations of Graafian follicle growth to ovulation in women using ultrasonic, laparoscopic and biochemical measurements. Br J Obstet Gynaec 88: 81–90, 1981.

17. Minoura S, Hara K, Okai T, et al: Ultrasonographic diagnosis of ovarian tumors. Proceedings of the 33rd Meeting of the Japan Society of Ultrasonics in Medicine, 1978, pp. 173–174.

20

DIFFERENTIATION OF BENIGN AND MALIGNANT LESIONS IN THE PANCREAS BY INTRAOPERATIVE ULTRASONIC IMAGING

Rod J. Lane

The pancreas is a regular source of frustration to the surgeon. The malignant disease processes affecting this gland commonly are not recognized until late, and even those discovered early, which may have some possibility of cure, are difficult to define pathologically, despite advances in transcutaneous imaging systems such as ultrasound (1, 2), endoscopic retrograde cholangiopancreatography (ERCP) (3, 4) and computerized axial tomography (5). Even after the surgeon exposes the mass, diagnosis may be difficult (6). Biopsying the gland has a small but definite morbidity (7), and regardless of the technique used, the false-negative biopsy rate is 15% (8). This problem is primarily due to sampling errors related to pancreatitis surrounding many malignant pancreatic lesions.

The correct identification of malignant lesions is important because resection carries the only hope of cure. A 40% 5-year survival rate is achieved with periampullary carcinomas, whereas with those arising from the acini, the prognosis is very poor (9). Yet, the mortality for pancreaticoduodenal resection is 5–20% (10) and, therefore, is not embarked upon lightly. A palliative bypass procedure, on the other hand, carries a relatively low morbidity rate, with the result that many surgeons perform this procedure without having adequately assessed pathology or resectability in the case of an early neoplasm. To misdiagnose a benign lesion and wrongly proceed to pancreatic resection, considering the high mortality rate, is as bad as leaving a potentially curable lesion in situ. There is no infallible algorithm for managing a mass in the head of the pancreas, but operative ultrasound is potentially helpful in two ways: in directing the biopsy needle away from perineoplastic inflammatory tissue and in indicating management directly by aiding in the differentiation of benign and malignant disease processes.

272

A

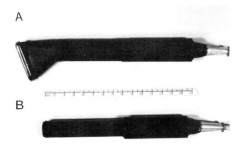

B

Figure 1. Two specifically designed operative probes (Cooper Medical Devices, Mountain View, California). In the probe shown in *A*, a small water path is provided to increase the scanning field close to the probe. Longer areas of the pancreas can be rapidly scanned. (*B*) Very small probe for areas of limited access.

With the introduction of smaller, mobile real-time systems, operative ultrasonic imaging is gaining recognition for its usefulness in detecting and differentiating lesions that the surgeon has difficulty palpating (11, 12). Further advances in intraoperative imaging have been made possible by specifically designed, sterilizable immersion operative probes that can be placed on the pancreas with ease (Figure 1). In addition, digital scan convertors are now available in the operative systems and they have made possible rather dramatic improvement in grey-scale imaging as well as freeze-frame facilities.

We have used operative ultrasonic imaging in 150 patients to assess the ultrasonic differences of normal, abnormal, benign and malignant processes in the pancreas. Also, because the surgeon may have difficulty in assessing resectability of a malignant lesion by palpation (usually determined by portal vein infiltration), an important secondary objective has been to assess local venous invasion.

METHOD

Optimal scans are produced when the ultrasonic probes are placed directly on the pancreatic parenchyma. In scanning the entire pancreas, the lesser sac is opened and the body and tail are exposed. In disease entities confined to the head of the gland, Kockerization of the duodenum is not required because the common bile duct and pancreatic head can be adequately shown by placing the probe on the duodenum itself (Figure 2). The head is examined initially by scanning parallel to the common bile duct, sphincter, portal vein and in-

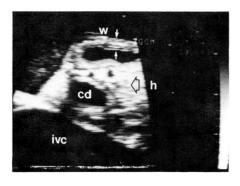

Figure 2. Cross section of head of a normal pancreas. (W) Duodenal wall; (cd) common bile duct. The pancreatic head (h) is in front of the inferior vena cava (ivc).

ferior vena cava. The origin of the superior mesenteric artery is assessed at this time. These sections intersect with the main and secondary pancreatic ducts in cross sections, which can then be traced to the tail of the gland with the splenic vessels, also in cross section. This allows easier location of the longitudinal section of the main pancreatic duct, which can be traced from the tail to the head of the gland with the splenic vessels running parallel posteriorly. The splenic vein moves with respiration and it may be necessary to have the anesthetist minimize respiratory excursion to facilitate scanning.

Acoustic coupling is achieved by moistening the surface of the gland with normal saline or, if difficulties arise because of insufficient contact, a sterile ultrasonic gel. Gel has been used in many cases without negative effect.

PATIENTS

We have seen 46 patients with some form of pancreatic mass enlargement or known pancreatic disease. In 39 cases we were confident of the diagnosis before operation. The cases of acute pancreatitis were diagnosed by laparotomy or encountered in the course of a routine cholecystectomy several weeks after the patients had come to us with gallstone pancreatitis. There were two cases of traumatic pancreatitis. The cases of chronic pancreatitis commonly were encountered in the course of routine cholecystectomy, particularly in elderly people with a mass in the head of the pancreas or, specifically, when some operative intervention was required for chronic pain in patients with known chronic pancreatitis. In each of these cases, preoperative ERCP had been performed.

Three benign neoplasms were found, two insulinomas and one gastrinoma. The malignant tumors consisted of 19 carcinomas of the head of the pancreas and one periampullary tumor. The majority of these advanced tumors were locally fixed or had metastasized to the liver, lymph nodes or peritoneum.

SURGICAL AND ULTRASONIC FINDINGS

In acute pancreatitis or acute resolving pancreatitis, the pancreas was macroscopically enlarged and edematous, and the main ducts were impalpable. Ultrasonographically, the primary and secondary ducts appeared dilated, as shown in Figure 3, and there were areas of decreased echogenicity, representing edema. Enlargement was generally uniform and symmetrical, except in traumatic pancreatitis, where the disruption of the parenchyma was replaced by large hypoechoic spaces representing hematoma and "leaked" pancreatic fluid.

In chronic pancreatitis, a much more variable ultrasonic picture was obtained. In focal lesions encountered in the elderly incidentally during cholecystectomy, the head of the gland was enlarged and indurated on palpation. Ultrasonographically, the primary ducts often appeared uniformly dilated, with the parenchyma showing areas of variable increased echogenicity representing fibrosis. In more florid cases, there sometimes was irregularity of

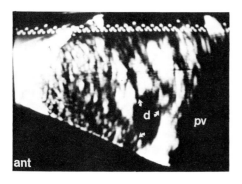

Figure 3. The main pancreatic duct (d) dilated in pancreatitis. The arrows indicate the origins of the secondary ducts. (pv) Portal vein system; (ant) anterior.

the bile and pancreatic ducts with multiple stenoses within one duct (Figure 4), atrophy of the parenchyma, areas of focal calcification and shadowing due to fat necrosis with asymmetrical, irregular enlargement. At operation very severe peripancreatic inflammation sometimes was found, such that without the ultrasonic images it would have been impossible to identify the pancreas as an anatomically distinct structure.

Benign tumors ultrasonically are like benign tumors elsewhere, but intraoperatively their features become very obvious. They tend to be very well circumscribed and symmetrically uniform in ultrasonic characteristics (unless some secondary degenerative changes have occurred) and tend to push and compress surrounding structures rather than invade and infiltrate, as malignant processes tend to do. This is illustrated in Figure 5, which shows a small insulinoma not located correctly by any transcutaneous technique. In Figure 5B, the solid arrows indicate the tumor pushing the parenchyma symmetrically into the splenic vein in longitudinal section. The open arrow indicates some local dilation of secondary ducts.

Malignant processes behave very differently, which shows up well ultrasonographically. The internal echoes usually are nonuniform and hypoechoic (Figure 6A). The borders are irregular and tend to infiltrate, particularly vessels such as the bile ducts and portal vein (Figure 6B). Pseudopods of tumor are readily identifiable. The posterior detail is poorly demonstrated, such that the surgeon finds himself increasing the gain to demonstrate posterior-lying structures. Although there are exceptions, malignant tumors tend to produce high attenuation. A summary of the common operative ultrasonic characteristics of pancreatic masses is given in Table 1.

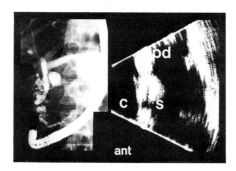

Figure 4. The pancreatic duct (pd) in a patient with chronic pancreatitis shows irregular dilatation and focal calcification (c), with shadowing posteriorly. (ant) Anterior.

TABLE 1. Mass in the Head of the Pancreas (at 10 MHz)

	Primary Ducts	Secondary Ducts	Parenchyma	Borders	Posterior details
Acute, Resolving Pancreatitis	Uniformly dilated in the mass	Dilated	Hypoechoic	Regular	Normal
Chronic Pancreatitis	Multiple stenosis in a single duct Uniform dilatation in the mass Secondary stones and calcification	Dilated or normal	Diffuse echogenic areas, areas of calcification and shadowing Atrophy	Varied, sometimes irregular	Normal, slightly higher gain may be required
Tumor (benign)	Normal	Some local dilatation	Hypoechoic	Regular	Normal, may be some through transmission
Tumor (malignant)	Obliterated, irregular infiltration, uniform distal dilation	Destroyed and obliterated	Hypoechoic	Very irregular	Difficult to image, high attenuation High gain required

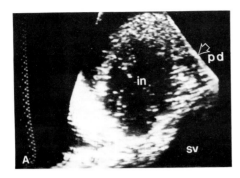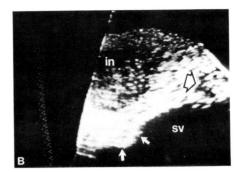

Figure 5. (A) Cross section of insulinoma (in) with pancreatic duct (pd) and splenic vein in cross section (sv). (B) Longitudinal section of insulinoma (in). The filled arrows (A) indicate pushing of the tumor into the splenic vein (sv). The open arrow (B) indicates some locally dilated secondary pancreatic ducts.

Seven patients presented difficulty at operation. Four were jaundiced pre-operatively, yet routine preoperative studies were equivocal. Two other patients were encountered at laparotomy for known pathology in another organ, and one patient had recurrent epigastric pain and a mass revealed by computerized tomography. Of the jaundiced patients, one presented with pancreatitis and no stones in the gallbladder and an ERCP showing a dilated pancreatic duct. The bile duct was not imaged. At operation there was a mass in the head of the pancreas but no stones in the gallbladder. Ultrasonic imaging showed a stone in the lower end of the common bile duct that eventually was removed: an unnecessary radical resection was avoided. Another three jaundiced patients were shown by ERCP to have multiple stenoses at the lower end of the common duct, and laparotomy showed a mass in the head of the pancreas. Two of these lesions were benign and one malignant, shown correctly by ultrasound. (The patient showing malignancy had a positive biopsy; the other two were alive and well after a bypass procedure 1 year later). The three remaining patients showed benign lesions on ultrasound and were alive and

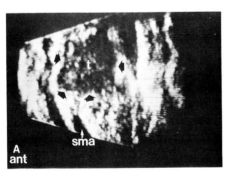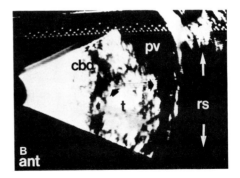

Figure 6. (A) Hypoechoic tumor (t) with irregular borders. (sma) Superior mesenteric artery; (ant) anterior. (B) Tumor (t) of the head of the pancreas infiltrating the common bile duct (cbd) and portal vein (pv). A relative shadow (rs) is created by the high attenuation produced by the tumor.

well 1 year later. Although the situation is relatively rare, operative ultrasound imaging was of great value in these particular cases, despite the use of relatively primitive equipment.

The technique has specific advantages to the surgeon over other procedures that are available at operation. Operative pancreatography has always been difficult to perform, particularly because of its invasive nature. The cannulation of the sphincter via duodenotomy has its own morbidity and is therefore unpopular. In addition, only the ducts are imaged. A comparison of the two techniques is shown in Table 2. Operative pancreatography is now approaching obsolescence.

Operative ultrasound imaging can also be used to assess the resectability of early pancreatic neoplasms by revealing portal vein invasion (Figure 6*B*). This is usually the factor that determines curability. However, early portal vein infiltration is difficult to palpate through the head of the pancreas and duodenum, and, thus, in the past if the lesion appeared resectable, a trial dissection was performed. Transcutaneous ultrasound can reveal advanced portal vein infiltration, but such infiltration is obvious at the time of operation. In early cases, the tumor itself may not be imaged, to say nothing of minimal portal vein infiltration (13). We have seen 16 cases in which the portal vein was scanned and a trial dissection carried out. Six appeared clinically resectable, but four of the six were shown by ultrasound imaging to have portal vein infiltration, which was confirmed by trial dissection. In one case the surgeon

TABLE 2.   Comparison of Operative Pancreaticosonography and Operative Pancreatography

	Operative Pancreaticosonography	Operative Pancreatography
Logistics	Noninvasive	Requires cannulation of pancreatic duct
Contrast	Not required	Contraindicated in contrast-allergic patients
Time	Complete scan, 5 min	Time-consuming, due to cannulation
Display	Parenchyma, ducts, portal vein	Ducts only, not beyond total obstructions
Repeatibility	1,800 images/min, real time	Static films only
Safety	Completely safe, even in pregnancy	Uses ionizing irradiation
Cost	Capital, similar to mobile x-ray unit Running costs, low	Similar capital costs Running costs much greater
User	Surgeon	Radiographer
Learning period	Operation, short Interpertation, long	Intemediate
Complications	None	Pancreatitis, fistula

TABLE 3.   Comparison of Operative Ultrasound and Transcutaneous Ultrasound

	Operative Ultrasound	Transcutaneous Ultrasound
Frequency	10–15 MHz	2.25–3.5 MHz
Resolution	Axial, 0.3–0.5 mm	1–2 mm
Intervening gaseous structures	Can be removed from field	May inhibit imaging
Organ location	Probe is placed directly on surface	May be difficult to scan entire region
Primary ducts	Routinely imaged	May be difficult to locate
Secondary ducts	Routinely imaged if dilated	Rarely seen
Attenuation characteristics of parenchyma	Relatively high related with higher frequency	Lower
Surrounding structures	Minor deformities in portal veins and biliary trees detected	Deformities visualized in advanced cases only

did not believe the ultrasonic findings, proceeded beyond the point of no return in the resection of the tumor and as a result was forced to resect a portion of the superior mesenteric vein.

As compared with transcutaneous techniques, operative ultrasound imaging has several advantages that are related primarily to the immediate proximity of the organ to the ultrasonic probe and the resultant high resolution. These features are compared in Table 3. In the intraoperative differentiation of benign and malignant processes, dilated secondary ducts in a sonolucent pancreas is the single most important feature. Transcutaneously, an area of decreased echogenicity can represent localized pancreatitis or tumor, and they commonly coexist (14). The resolution of the transcutaneous technique is not sufficient to allow differentiation of these diseases.

In conclusion, although intraoperative ultrasonography of the pancreas is in its infancy and surgeons are generally inexperienced in ultrasonic imaging, there appear to be ultrasonic characteristics that will aid in solving some of the problems that confront the surgeon operating on this difficult organ.

REFERENCES

1. Arger PH, Mulhern CG, Benavita JA, et al: An analysis of pancreatic sonography in suspected pancreatic disease. J Clin Ultrasound 7: 91–97, 1979.
2. Wright CH, Maklad F, Rosenthal SJ: Grey-scale ultrasonic characteristics of carcinoma of the pancreas. Br J Radiol 52: 281–288, 1979.
3. Mackie CR, Cooper MJ, Lewis MH, et al: Non-operative differentiation between pancreatic cancer and chronic pancreatitis. Ann Surg 189: 480–487, 1979.

4. Cotton PB, Lees WR, Vallon AG et al: Grey-scale ultrasonography and endoscopic pancreatography in pancreatic diagnosis. Radiology 134: 453–459, 1980.

5. Whalen JP: Impact of new imaging methods. Am J Radiology 133: 585–618, 1979.

6. Gmeco MB, Braasch JW, Rossi RL: Mass in the head of the pancreas. Surg Clin North Am 60: 333–347, 1980.

7. Schultz NJ, Sanders RJ: Evaluation of pancreatic biopsy. Ann Surg 158: 1053–1057, 1963.

8. Hermann RE: Manual of Surgery of the Gallbladder, Bile Ducts and Exocrine Pancreas. Comprehensive Manuals of Surgical Specialties. New York, Springer-Verlag, 1979.

9. Warren KW, Veidenheimer MC, Pratt HS: Pancreatoduodenectomy for periampullary cancer. Surg Clin North Am 47: 639–645, 1967.

10. Braasch JW, Gray BN: Considerations that lower pancreatoduodenectomy mortality. Am J Surg 133: 480–484, 1977.

11. Lane RJ, Coupland GAE: Ultrasonic indications to explore the common bile duct. Surgery 91: 268–274, 1982.

12. Coelho JCU, Sigel B, Flanigan DP, et al: An experimental evaluation of arteriography and imaging ultrasonography in detecting arterial defects at operation. J Surg Res 32: 130–137, 1982.

13. Ariyama J, Shirakabe H, Ikenabe H, et al: The diagnosis of the small resectable pancreatic carcinoma. Clin Radiol 28: 437–444, 1977.

14. Leopold G: Echographic study of the pancreas. JAMA 232: 287–289, 1975.

III
Future Prospects

21

PROSPECTS FOR ULTRASOUND IN TUMOR DIAGNOSIS

George Kossoff

The imaging capabilities of static and real-time B-mode equipment have been dramatically improved in the last 10 years. Today, the standard of performance is very good and is beginning to approach theoretical limits. Indeed, today echograms obtained with different equipment from the same patient bear close resemblance, suggesting that a plateau in performance has been attained. This means not only that poor quality equipment no longer is on the market but also that advances will be more difficult to achieve in the future. Undoubtedly, improvements will continue to be made as physicists better understand the laws of propagation of ultrasound and engineers apply more fully the principles of communication theory made possible by advances in integrated circuit technology. These improvements must, however, be cost effective. It is possible, therefore, that they will be introduced slowly and that the imaging characteristics of current equipment will be the standard of performance for the next few years.

Future developments in ultrasound are likely to come from a number of areas. It is most likely that new clinical areas will make use of existing instrumentation. Special-purpose equipment using conventional technology is now appearing on the market, and this, too, could lead to new uses of ultrasound. Particularly promising in this regard is equipment that combines B-mode and pulsed Doppler techniques and is capable of measuring blood flow to major organs. Improvements in the performance of conventional equipment will also influence future developments because they will improve the accuracy of established techniques and allow new measurements. Finally, the ultimate potential of diagnostic ultrasound will be realized by the development of equipment capable of quantitative measurement of acoustic parameters of tissue. This will have an effect similar to that of computerized tomography in the field of radiology. Thus, the prospects for diagnostic ultrasound appear to be quite promising, and the method is unlikely to be replaced by other new developments in diagnostic technology, such as digital radiography and nuclear magnetic resonance.

NEW AREAS OF CLINICAL APPLICATION

In the past many new areas of clinical application have been developed by the use of existing instrumentation in new ways. The use of ultrasonography to examine upper abdominal anatomy in the operating room is an example of a recently introduced technique. Now that the attention of surgeons has been drawn to this application, it is likely that ultrasound will be used in other, similar, situations. For example, intraoperative real-time echographic examination of the brain is being evaluated by neurosurgeons for the purpose of locating lesions, directing needle aspiration biopsies and decompressing cystic lesions (1). The technique has already been shown to be reliable and rapid, resulting in less exploratory surgery. The use of this technique to visualize small tumors is illustrated in Figure 1.

The use of contrast agents is an integral part of the practice of radiology. To date, no ultrasonic contrast agents have been developed to enhance the reflectivity of human tissues, but encouraging results have been obtained in animal experiments using aqueous solutions (2) and collagen microspheres (3). Presumably this work will encourage more studies, and the introduction of first-generation contrast agents must be considered a distinct possibility for the not-too-distant future.

The use of existing instrumentation in combination with other techniques is another area of potential development. For example, the use of ultrasound imaging to guide biopsy needles opened up a major new area of clinical application. The use of ultrasound techniques to assist the placement of radioactive pellets in soft tissue tumors could become another combined application.

SPECIAL-PURPOSE EQUIPMENT

Diagnostic ultrasound is now attracting the attention of many specialists, and special-purpose equipment designed to their requirements is beginning to appear on the market. Specially designed probes are being developed for use by surgeons in the operating room, and transrectal and transurethral scanners are being used by urologists. Real-time scanning is being introduced to internal scanners, and high-frequency probes are being evaluated for use in conjunction with endoscopes. Ultrasound imaging has the potential to demonstrate sub-

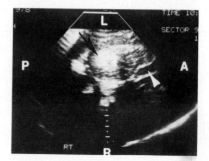

Figure 1. Axial real-time echogram obtained in the operating room showing a spherical echogenic mass (black arrow) that proved to be a grade II astrocytoma on needle biopsy. The ventricle (white arrow) is also visualized (courtesy of T. M. Silver, and James Knake, University of Michigan).

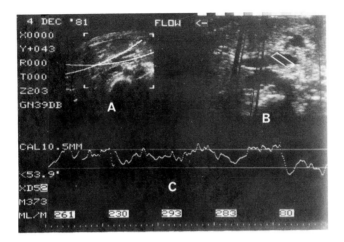

Figure 2. (A) Scan of the upper abdomen showing various abdominal vessels. (B) Close-up of boxed area with Doppler sample volume positioned over splenic vein. (C) Quantitative print-out of volume of blood flow in splenic vein.

mucosal structures, and this could encourage gastroenterologists to utilize the method.

Equipment based on the combined use of B-mode and pulsed Doppler techniques that allows the quantitative measurement of blood flow (4, 5) is likely to prove very important for the ultrasonic diagnosis of cancer. The measurement is performed as follows. The vessel of interest is identified on the B-mode image and its diameter and orientation are noted. The pulsed Doppler sample is then placed so as to encompass the vessel and used to measure the average velocity of blood in the vessel. From these parameters, the instantaneous blood flow is derived and plotted on the screen, as illustrated in Figure 2. At present, the method is most suitable for measurement of blood flow in vessels ranging in diameter from 4 to 10 mm and in which the peak velocity is less than 150 cm/s. The veins and arteries of the major upper abdominal organs generally satisfy these requirements. A potential application lies in the evaluation of splenic blood flow in generalized involvements, such as leukemia, and renal blood flow as affected by tumors. In this application, the ability to measure flow in the contralateral organ should allow the detection of a relatively small change in blood flow caused by the tumor.

IMPROVEMENTS IN EQUIPMENT PERFORMANCE

Most of the equipment on the market today was designed to optimize the display of the low-level echoes obtained from the internal structure of tissues when examined in the simple scan mode. Because of their many advantages, digital scan converters are much used, and considerable research is devoted to improving the quality of digital echograms and to provide investigators with the advantages to be gained from instruments with the capability of storing echograms in digital memory. These efforts will undoubtedly be rewarded, and in the near future echograms should lose their digital appearance and surpass the quality of analogue scans.

Equipment generally is not designed for the display of strong echoes inasmuch as these are generally compressed or saturated into the top of the grey scale display range. For this reason, air and calcifications, which are readily distinguished by radiology, are difficult to identify ultrasonically. With current equipment, both are portrayed as a strong anterior echo with pronounced shadowing. Careful attention to the subtle aspects of the echograms can in some instances allow the distinction (6). An air interface reflects all of the incident energy. It therefore is more likely to give rise to multiple reflections while the strength of the echo lifts the ringing that follows into the displayed range. Thus, somewhat anomalously on preliminary consideration, the shadow behind the air interface is not as pronounced or clean as that behind calcifications. Improved performance of equipment that allows distinction between the amplitudes of strong echoes should allow this differentiation.

Simple scanning has many advantages in the provision of ultrasonic images. The echograms may be formed using few lines of sight and therefore acquired in real time. The echograms readily portray small changes in the attenuating properties by signs such as enhancement or shadowing of posterior detail. Finally, the textural representation of the internal structure of soft tissues is not degraded by the lack of superposition of echoes due to small variations in the velocity of propagation in the tissues. To remove the effect of the variable manual scanning speed of the static scanner, peak detect signal processing is universally employed. This form of signal processing is the most economical to implement on digital scan converters and is also employed in real-time equipment.

Compound scanning has been underutilized so far. The method has certain advantages, such as the more complete portrayal of boundaries of structures. It also is more suitable for the acquisition of whole-body scans. These more clearly illustrate anatomical relationships, which sometimes are difficult to appreciate on the limited "keyhole" views obtained with real-time equipment. The textural representation of soft tissue structure obtained on compound scans is less prone to the speckle artifact typical of simple scans, and it is not always appreciated that this textural representation is complementary to that obtained with simple scanning.

The nature of reflections from interfaces is a function of their geometry. In diagnostic investigations these range from specular reflections originating from large structures to diffuse reflections from small structures. With compound scanning, structures are examined from many different directions, from which they may return echoes of differing magnitude. It therefore is possible to utilize different types of signal processing techniques to select the portrayal of the desired ratio of specular and diffuse echoes and thus optimize the display of desired detail (7).

With peak detection, the maximum value of an echo is displayed. Specular reflectors return a strong echo only from one direction and compound scanning in combination with this method of detection ensures that this value of echo is displayed, i.e., the method optimizes the portrayal of specular echoes. Unfortunately, the beamwidth echoes are also displayed at full strength, and areas of low reflectivity lying close to strong reflectors are readily obscured.

In the integrate detection mode the sum of the echoes originating from an area equal to one pixel in the digital image is displayed. Average detect is an alternate, similar, method in which the displayed magnitude is obtained by dividing the sum by the number of times the pixel has been updated. Inasmuch as specular reflectors give rise to a strong echo from one direction only and diffuse reflectors give rise to the same echo from all directions, integrate and average detect emphasize the display of diffuse echoes. By emphasizing the central echo, the integrate and average detect reduce the effective beamwidth, thus improving the spatial resolution. Also, the speckle effect seen on simple scans and peak-detected compound scans is replaced by a more even texture, allowing better appreciation of small variations in grey scale, i.e., an improvement in contrast resolution is also attained. The difference in appearance obtained with peak and average detect is illustrated in Figure 3. The echograms are of a patient with a large hepatoma. Because of the improved spatial resolution, the gallbladder and the small vessels in the liver are more clearly displayed on the average detect image. The improvement in the contrast resolution may be appreciated by noting the uniform liver texture and the reduced echogenicity of the involved areas in the liver surrounding the gallbladder.

Minimum detect is another form of signal processing. It is the reverse of the peak detect method in that after the first simple scan has been stored, the minimum value of the echoes from the following scans is retained. Specular reflectors are therefore displayed by their minimum value and are thus effectively removed from the display. Being essentially a subtractive technique, the method also emphasizes the display of echo-free areas. The potential applications are the improved visualization of microcalcifications and of ducts, features of interest in the diagnostic evaluation of the breast. An example of

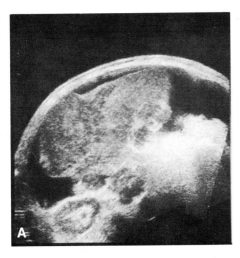 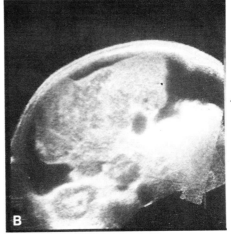

Figure 3. Peak (*A*) and average (*B*) detect echograms of patient with a large hepatoma.

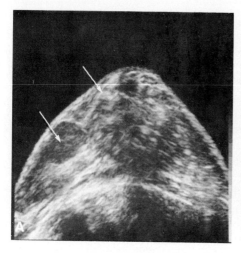 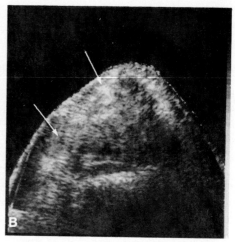

Figure 4. Peak (A) and minimum (B) detect echograms of patient with a large fibroadenoma and prominent diffuse reflector.

the peak and minimum detect processes is illustrated in Figure 4. The peak-detected image clearly portrays a fibroadenoma encapsulated by boundary echoes. The pectoralis muscle layers are also visualized. These specular reflectors are removed in the minimum detect echogram, which shows a prominent diffuse reflector lying in the anterior portion of the breast. Because of the presence of other specular reflectors in that portion of the breast, the diffuse reflector is not as readily perceived on the peak-detected echogram.

QUANTIFIED MEASUREMENT OF ACOUSTIC PARAMETERS

Ultrasonography today can reveal tumors with a specificity in the high 80% range and a sensitivity in the mid-90% range. This is impressive when one considers that this diagnostic technique is based on the qualitative assessment of only one acoustic parameter of tissue, namely, the acoustic impedance discontinuity and the indirect portrayal of a second parameter, attenuation, by signs such as shadowing or enhancement. The third acoustic parameter, Doppler, has been used for some time for the study of flow and for imaging but has not been used for cancer diagnosis. Of the information resident in the fourth parameter, echo-scattering cross section, only the directly back-reflected energy is employed. Velocity, the fifth parameter, is generally ignored and considered a degrading factor, because it smears the spatial resolution of compound scans. Finally, our incomplete appreciation of the laws of propagation and reflection of ultrasound does not allow the measurement of the sixth parameter, acoustic impedance, except under highly simplified experimental conditions. There is, therefore, considerable room for improvement through the development of techniques that would allow the quantitative measurement of these six independent acoustic parameters, their dependence on the nature of the interrogation beam, such as intensity and frequency, and on the physiological activity of the tissues. By comparison, it may be appropriate to note that the whole practice of radiology is based on the measurement of only one radiological parameter of tissue, the x-ray absorption coefficient.

Modern technical developments are closely linked to the employment of digital signal processing techniques, and it is highly likely that computers will play a central role in the attainment of advances in ultrasonic diagnosis. Computers are expensive, and their use will have to be justified by their cost effectiveness. It is important, therefore, to identify the major limitations of the simple B-mode technique and to determine what measurement of which acoustic parameter of tissue in which organ or clinical setting would best overcome these limitations. Further because of its effectiveness, the simple B-mode technique is likely to remain the primary ultrasonic examination procedure. It will continue to be used to identify areas of interest and to reveal geometrical relationships. Measurement of acoustic properties of tissues in a limited area with coarser resolution will allow less-powerful computers to be employed, making the measurement techniques more cost effective.

Although techniques for measuring acoustic parameters await development, some general statements may be made on their applicability. Measurement of amplitude of echoes provides information concerning acoustic impedance mismatch and forms the basis of the simple B-mode technique. Movement of echoes in response to the cardiac cycle or external vibrations could be used to determine the elasticity of tissues. Attenuation from echographic data may be measured by analysis of echo from a standard reflector behind the tissues of interest (8). This technique is possible only in the operating room where such a reflector can be introduced behind the surgically exposed tissues. Alternatively the measurement may be made by comparison of the frequency content of echoes received from near and distant reflectors (9). Attenuation may also be measured by transmission reconstruction techniques (10) similar to those employed in computerized tomography. Unfortunately, the breast is the only major organ that can be examined by this technique. Doppler techniques involve the measurement of the frequency shift of the signal caused by moving reflectors. Flowing blood can thus be considered to be a natural contrast agent in the body. Measurement of echo-scattering cross section requires the presence of reflectors and the ability to examine the tissues either from different directions or over a wide frequency range. The velocity of ultrasound may be measured by transmission reconstruction techniques. As with attenuation, the application of this technique is restricted to the breast.

It recently was shown that velocity measurements may also be performed by analysis of data obtained from a compound scan (11). The principle of the technique as applied to a two-velocity model is illustrated in Figure 5. The structure is scanned from one position and the simple scan echogram is stored in digital memory. If the velocity in the object differs from that in the coupling path, then, due to refraction, the ultrasonic beam is deflected and echoes are obtained from impedance discontinuities lying along the deflection path. The equipment, however, is unaware of this deviation and plots the echoes as though they were being obtained from the original line of sight. The structure is then examined from another position and the second scan is stored. Re-

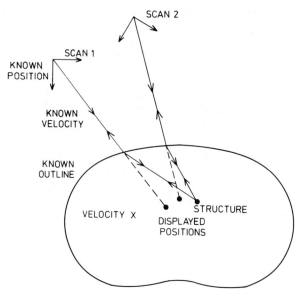

Figure 5. Schematic representation of principle used for measurement of velocity by cross correlation to superimpose position of structure obtained with two simple scans.

fraction again deflects the ultrasonic beam, but, because different lines of sight are employed, the echoes from the same impedance discontinuities are not plotted in the same position, i.e., they fail to superimpose. The technique relies on identifying the same structure on the two echograms and measuring the lack of superposition. This information, combined with the shape of the velocity boundary interface obtained from the B-mode image, is used to measure the velocity in the examined structure. The method has been applied to measure velocity in larger organs such as the liver. Two simple echograms portraying a duct used for determining the lack of superposition are shown in Figure 6. Comparison of results obtained at different depths and in different planes gave values of velocity for normal liver which averaged 1,575 m/s with a variation of less than 15 m/s, suggesting that the method may be used to measure velocity to an accuracy of 1%. Studies are being undertaken to develop the technique to allow measurement of velocity in a number of organs with different velocities, and, if successful, would represent a major advance in diagnostic ultrasound.

Some of the limitations of the simple B-mode technique that potentially are amenable to ultrasonic diagnosis lie in the following areas:

1. Identification of different types of biological liquids. Homogeneous liquids such as urine, free blood and ascites are displayed as echo-free areas. They, therefore, cannot be distinguished by the acoustic impedance mismatch. Since no internal echoes are present, attenuation, Doppler and echo-scattering cross section measurements cannot be performed. Due to the varying protein and salt content, the velocity in these liquids differs by a few per-

cent and a velocity measurement technique with sufficient accuracy to distinguish these variations could be used to perform the identification.

2. Differentiation between cystic and solid masses when these contain low-level echoes. Cystic lesions that contain debris or particulate matter, such as abscesses, are sometimes difficult to distinguish from poorly echogenic solid tumors, such as lymphomas. The velocity in liquids is generally several percent less than that in soft tissues, and velocity measurement techniques can potentially allow the differentiation. Experimental data are necessary to determine whether this is the most sensitive parameter or whether measurement of attenuation is preferable. Another avenue is the study of small movement in tissue in response to the cardiac cycle. It is possible that the elastic forces in tissue will cause a regular pattern of movement of echoes from within soft tissues, whereas the movement of echoes within cystic lesions will be more random. The use of externally induced vibrations to enhance such movements could be useful for the differentiation.

3. Distinction of fat from other soft tissues. Fat has unusual acoustic properties in that subcutaneous fat within the breast is essentially nonechogenic, whereas in the orbit and deep within the body it is strongly echogenic. The identification of fat is particularly important in the breast, where malignant tumors are portrayed as similar relatively echo-free areas. Although the attenuation of fat is generally less than that of other soft tissues, its most characteristic acoustic feature is the very slow velocity of propagation, and the development of even a relatively coarse velocity measurement technique should allow the distinction of fat from other soft tissues.

4. Determination of degree of involvement by disseminated processes. Currently disseminated processes are identified by noting the change in the relative reflectivity of adjacent organs, the subjective assessment of change in attenuation and difference in appearance of secondary signs, such as

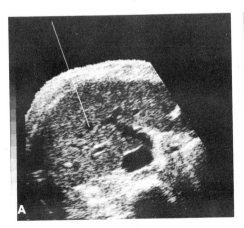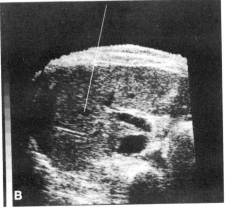

Figure 6.   Two simple scans portraying duct used for cross correlation superimposition.

degree of prominence of portal radicles in the liver. Many disseminated conditions are characterized by changes associated with increased fibrosis and fatty infiltration. These cause the velocity and attenuation to increase and decrease respectively, and development of relatively accurate measurement techniques of these two parameters complemented by information from echo-scattering cross section measurement should allow the quantitative determination of infiltrative processes.

5. Assessment of degree of vascularity of tumors. Doppler ultrasound recently has been applied to detect the extra blood flow associated with rapidly growing tumors in the breast, in particular around the periphery of the lesions (12). There is no theoretical reason why the method could not be extended to measure the total blood volume of vascularized tissue, thus allowing assessment of the functional requirements of tumors.

6. Distinction among and identification of normal, benign and malignant tissues. This histological identification represents the ultimate aim. It could be achieved for many tissues by the quantitative measurement of all six acoustic parameters of tissue. This goal also includes the detection of premalignant changes in tissue, which could be identified by ultrasonic recognition of hyperplastic changes. This would open up the whole area of screening to ultrasound examination. For example, it is thought that premalignant changes in the breast manifest themselves by relatively general enlargement of ductal and lobular structure with epithelial cell proliferation (13). These changes reach dimensions that potentially could be revealed by ultrasound, opening the possibility of screening the breast for precancerous changes.

CONCLUSION

Diagnostic ultrasound has reached the stage of relative maturity in that the static and real-time B-mode equipment has plateaued at a high standard level of performance. The method is based on the qualitative assessment of only one acoustic parameter of tissue, acoustic impedance discontinuity, and indirect portrayal of a second parameter, attenuation. Tissues may be assessed by measurement of six independent acoustic parameters, and diagnostic ultrasound will not achieve its full potential until techniques are developed that will allow the qualitative measurement of all these parameters. Although it is difficult to estimate the impact that these techniques will have, there is no doubt that significant clinical advances will be achieved and that the prospects of tumor diagnosis by ultrasound are most promising.

REFERENCES

1. Knake JE, Silver TM, Chandler WF: Intraoperative cranial sonography for neurosurgical procedures. Semin Ultrasound (in press).
2. Ophir J, McWhirt RE, Malclad NF: Aqueous solutions as potential ultrasonic contrast agents. Ultrasonic Imaging 1: 265–279, 1979.

3. Ophir J, Gobuty A, McWhirt RE, et al: Ultrasonic backscatter from contrast producing collagen microspheres. Ultrasonic imaging 2: 67–77, 1980.

4. Gill RW, Trudinger BJ, Garrett WJ, et al: Fetal umbilical venous flow measured in utero by pulsed Doppler and B-mode ultrasound in normal pregnancies. Am J Obstet Gynecol 139: 720–725, 1981.

5. Gill RW, Warren PS: Blood flow measurement using pulsed Doppler and B-mode ultrasound. Principles and applications. Ultrasonics 2: 279–287, 1981.

6. Sommer FG, Taylor KJ: Differentiation of acoustic shadowing due to calculi and gas collections. Radiology 135: 399–403, 1980.

7. Robinson DE, Knight PC: Computer reconstruction techniques in compound scan pulse echo imaging. Ultrasonic Imaging 3: 217–234, 1981.

8. Robinson DE: Computer Spectral Analysis of Ultrasound A-Mode Echoes in Utrasonic Tissue Characterisation. II. In Linzer M (Ed): NBS Special Publication 525. Washington DC, US Government Printing Office, 281–286.

9. Kuc R: Clinical application of an ultrasound co-efficient estimation technique for liver pathology characterisation. IEEE Trans Biomed Eng 27: 1980, 312–319.

10. Greenleaf JF, Bahn RC: Clinical imaging with transmissive ultrasonic computerised tomography. IEEE Trans Biomed Eng 28: 177–185, 1981.

11. Robinson DE, Chen F, Wilson LS: Measurement of velocity of propagation from ultrasonic pulse echo data. Ultrasound Med Biol (in press).

12. Burns PN, Halliwell M, Wells PNT: Ultrasonic Doppler studies of the breast. Ultrasound Med Biol (in press).

13. Wellings SR, Jansen HM, Marami RG: Atlas of subgross pathology of the human breast with special reference to possible precancerous lesions. J Nat Cancer Inst 55: 231–273, 1975.

INDEX